HEPATITIS B VIRUS AND IMMUNE RESPONSE

S. FIORINO, R. VUKOTIC, E. LOGGI,
G. VITALE, C. CURSARO, A. GRAMENZI,
L. MICCO, C. FORTINI, A. CUPPINI,
M. BERNARDI AND P. ANDREONE

Nova Science Publishers, Inc.

New York

For permission to use material from this book please contact us:
Telephone 631-231-7269; Fax 631-231-8175
Web Site: http://www.novapublishers.com

NOTICE TO THE READER

The Publisher has taken reasonable care in the preparation of this book, but makes no expressed or implied warranty of any kind and assumes no responsibility for any errors or omissions. No liability is assumed for incidental or consequential damages in connection with or arising out of information contained in this book. The Publisher shall not be liable for any special, consequential, or exemplary damages resulting, in whole or in part, from the readers' use of, or reliance upon, this material. Any parts of this book based on government reports are so indicated and copyright is claimed for those parts to the extent applicable to compilations of such works.

Independent verification should be sought for any data, advice or recommendations contained in this book. In addition, no responsibility is assumed by the publisher for any injury and/or damage to persons or property arising from any methods, products, instructions, ideas or otherwise contained in this publication.

This publication is designed to provide accurate and authoritative information with regard to the subject matter covered herein. It is sold with the clear understanding that the Publisher is not engaged in rendering legal or any other professional services. If legal or any other expert assistance is required, the services of a competent person should be sought. FROM A DECLARATION OF PARTICIPANTS JOINTLY ADOPTED BY A COMMITTEE OF THE AMERICAN BAR ASSOCIATION AND A COMMITTEE OF PUBLISHERS.

Library of Congress Cataloging-in-Publication Data

Hepatitis B virus and immune response / S. Fiorino ... [et al.] (authors).
   p. ; cm.
Includes bibliographical references and index.
ISBN 978-1-60456-450-1 (hardcover)
1. Hepatitis B virus. 2. Hepatis B--Immunological aspects. I. Fiorino, S. (Sirio)
[DNLM: 1. Hepatitis B virus--immunology. 2. Hepatitis B Antibodies--immunology. 3. Immunity, Cellular. QW 170 H5288 2008]
QR201.H46H442 2008
616.3'623--dc22
                              2008011191

Published by Nova Science Publishers, Inc. ✣ New York

HEPATITIS B VIRUS AND IMMUNE RESPONSE

DATE DUE

Contents

Chapter I

Introduction

Hepatitis B virus (HBV) is a small DNA virus, that may cause both acute and chronic liver damage. Wide evidence suggests that age in which HBV is acquired influences strongly the outcome of infection [1]. Whereas approximately 90-95% of acutely HBV-infected immunocompetent adults experience a self-limiting hepatitis with the establishment of a protective long-lasting immunity, the remaining 5-10% develop a chronic hepatitis with different patterns of severity and course. About 400 million people [2] in the world present a chronic HBV infection, an important cause of cirrhosis, hepatocellular carcinoma and liver failure [3,4,5]. Neonatal transmission of HBV causes an higher rate of chronic infection, approximately 90% of infected children become chronic carriers. Viral and host factors causing HBV persistence are not completely understood, although in the last years a large series of studies have evaluated factors and mechanisms involved in HBV unsuccessful clearance. It is widely accepted that this virus is not directly cytopathic for hepatocytes. Liver is rather related to cell-mediated immunity and inflammation [6,7]. Resolution of acute HBV hepatitis requires strong, polyclonal and multispecific HLA class I and II restricted CD4+ and CD8+ T cell responses to viral envelope, nucleocapsid and polymerase determinants. In patients with chronic infection, immune response is shown to be defective or undetectable and consequently unuseful in HBV control and eradication [8]. Although mechanisms involved in inflammatory and immune response in acute and chronic HBV infections have been extensively studied, several questions remain unsolved. Moreover, in the last years several key steps in research have contributed to improve our present knowledge of immunopathogenesis of HBV infection [9].

With reference to studies performed in vitro, animals and humans, the following points are discussed in this review :

1. Normal immunitary system function during viral infections ;
2. HBV gcnome organization;
3. HBV antigens and epitopes modulating lymphocyte subsets immune response in peripheral blood and liver tissue;
4. Cytokines and growth factors induced in the host by viral antigens, during HBV acute or chronic infection;
5. Immune response mechanisms promoting HBV clearance or persistence with particular regard to adaptive immune response and activity of HBV-specific CD4+ and CD8+ T cells;
6. Immune response in HBV chronic infection under antiviral treatment with nucleotide or nucleoside analogues;
7. Possible mechanisms and events involved in immune response dysfunctions in HBV chronic infection.

Chapter II

Normal Immunitary System Response during Viral Infection

Immunological protection against viral infections is provided both by innate and adaptive responses [10]. The former arm of immune system includes complement, phagocytes and natural killer cells, the latter consists of antigen-presenting cells, macrophages, B-lymphocytes, plasma cells and T lymphocytes [11]. In the last years several evidences contributed to improve and to modify previous understanding of immune response function. A specific and efficacious immune response against intracellular pathogens such as viruses requires a fine and tightly regulated interaction and cooperation in the context of a dynamic network among antigens, responding cells, cytokines and accessory molecules [12]. In this setting antigen-presenting cells, macrophages, B, T, NK and NKT cells act in cross-talk, modulating and influencing the maturation and function of one another [2]. Final immune response, in term of its magnitude, length and efficacy, depends both on reciprocal interplay among cells of immune system and on complex balance between their activating and inhibitory signals [13]. To date reports available are suggesting that liver is a lymphoid organ with particular immunological properties [14].

Antigen-Presenting Cells

The generation and development of an effective antigen-specific immune response needs proper interaction and cooperation between an effector cell, such as T lymphocyte, and an antigen-presenting cells (APCs) [15].

A wide variety of cells possess properties of APCs, including B cells, endothelial cells and macrophages, but only dendritic cells (DCs) are defined professional cells, according to their capability to activate very efficiently naïve T cells. These cells constitute the first line defense, controlling the surrounding microenvironment and immediately identifying the molecules associated with invading microorganisms, by means of diversified series of receptors [16]. Toll-like receptors (TLRs) constitute a sensing system with a key role in the recognition of different pathogens. To date 13 human TLRs have been detected, TLR2, TLR3, TLR4 and TLR9, are activated in response to double-stranded RNA viruses, whereas TLR7 and TLR8 are stimulated by single-stranded RNA viruses [17,18]. DCs are present in an immature resting state at sites potentially accessible to pathogens, scattered throughout non-lymphoid tissues. After binding of TLRs with their proper antigen, DCs are activated and undergo a differentiation program to become mature effector cells. Several key steps are involved in this process [19,20], including:

- captation and processing of antigens, at periphery, by DCs, via endocytosis and proteolysis, with subsequent exposure, on their cellular surface, of generated-epitopes [21];
- homing of activated DCs via lymphatic vessels to T cell-rich areas of secondary lymphoid organs, such as lymph nodes. This migration is regulated by a wide variety of receptors, such as CCR7 [22]. Furhermore it is now accepted that some invading microorganisms may enter lymph nodes directly [23] and be captured by DCs in these sites;
- presentation of epitopes, loaded on cellular surface of DCs, to specific-antigen-T cells in association with both appropriate Major Histocompatibility Complex (MHC) restricted setting and with costimulatory molecules, represented by CD40, CD80 (B7-1), CD86 (B7-2), CD58 (LFA-3) and CD54 (ICAM-1) [24] ;

- proliferation and differentiation of naïve-T populations into cytotoxic or helper subsets with cytokine secreting abilities, following recognition of their specific antigens [25].

Cooperation between T helper cells and APCs induces activation of both B and T cytotoxic lymphocytes. At the end of this process naïve-B clones become secreting-plasma cells and T cytotoxic subsets may perform their effector function against infected target cells.

Specific-T helper cells recognize antigens in the context of MHC class II, whereas specific-cytotoxic T cells are activated, following encounter of protein-fragments exposed in the groove of APC-bound MHC I molecule. At least two different and distinct DCs populations have been detected in humans, with regard to their functional and morphological patterns: myeloid DCs (mDCs) and plasmacytoid DCs (pDCs) [26]. The former subset includes cells expressing CD11c/CD1b, TLR 1, 2, 3, 4, 5, 6 and 7 markers involved in antigen uptake, T cell stimulation and IL-12 release, the latter consists of cells exhibiting CD123 (IL-3R α-chain), TLR 6, 7, 8 and 9 and secreting TNF-α [27,28]. A fine and tightly regulated interplay involves T effector cells (with helper, regulatory and cytotoxic properties), DCs, natural killer and natural killer T cells, modulating the microenvironmental milieu and cytokine release, during the distinct phases of immune response [29,30]. It has been observed that IL-12 secretion by myeloid DCs after encounter with their ligand, promotes strong IFN-γ production by effector CD4 + T and NK cells [31]. Naive T helper cells also are induced to release IFN-γ, that drives these precursors to acquire a Th1 polarization. In addition to IL-12, also IL-23 and IL-27, all belonging to IL-12 family, have been reported to promote IFN-γ release, with different degree of efficiency [32]. Down-regulation of IL-12 family molecules production, in association with IL-4 release, secreted by T helper cell subsets themselves, induce naïve Th to acquire a Th2 phenotype [33]. According with their central role in immune system, DCs represent a bridge linking innate and adaptive immune response [34]. Mature DCs cells are considered as discrete packets of information to prime naïve T cells [13], because once they have migrated to lymph nodes have a finite short life: their survival is only few days long [35].

Natural Killer Cells

Natural killer (NK) population [36], in association with DCs, is an essential component of innate immune response and include a wide variety of lymphoid cells, representing about 5-10% of human peripheral blood mononuclear lymphocytes [37]. NKs possess the capacity to respond very rapidly after their activation and to kill spontaneously different cell lines via a major histocompatibility complex-restricted independent manner, without pre-sensitization [38]. Therefore they represent the first line of immunological defense direct against viral infection and neoplastic cells. On account of remarkable complexity of markers and functions displayed by NKs, the characterization of these cells is still incomplete and thus needs further investigations [39]. According to the expression of CD56 density, human NKs can be subdivided into CD56^{bright} and CD56^{dim} [40,41]. The majority of NKs show a CD56^{dim} phenotype in association with high levels of CD16, about 10% of NKs are CD56^{bright} and have low levels of CD16. The latter cells present the chemokine receptor 7 (CCR7) and CXC-chemokine receptor 3 (CXCR3), whereas the former express CXCR1 and CX3C-chemokine receptor 1 (CX3CR1) and are devoid of CCR7 [42,43]. CD56^{bright} NKs express a major cytotoxic activity in comparison to CD56^{dim} cells. It has been suggested that during a viral infection the NKs, by means of their activatory and inhibitory cellular surface receptors, recognize different molecules on their target cells, such as pathogen-encoded antigens, or self-proteins, which can be up- or down-regulated in viral infections [44]. The final effector functions exhibited by NKs result from dynamic and closely regulated balance of the series of signals acting on these cells [45]. Following their activation, NKs show two key properties: strong cytotoxic function against infected target cells, through cell to cell direct contact and secretion of a wide pattern of pro-inflammatory cytokines with anti-viral properties, such as IFN-γ, TNF-α, TNF-β, IL-3, G-CSF (granulocyte colony-stimulating factor) and M-CSF (macrophage colony-stimulating factor), IL-10 and IL-13 [46]. NKs and DCs exert their activity in concert, influencing reciprocally their maturation and modulating the magnitude and quality of innate and adaptive immune responses at different steps [47]. The presence of IL-12 or IL-4 induces NKs to secrete respectively IL-10 and IFN-γ or IL-5 and IL-13 [48]. NK-mediated killing of virus-infected target cells favours the release of viral molecules, which are captured by dendritic and antigen-presenting cells and then exposed on their cellular surface, improving the efficiency of epitopes presentation to specific lymphocytes [49]. In addition activated NKs, releasing different cytokines such as INF-γ, promote maturation of DCs, which acquire the abilities to secrete IL-12. The modulation of environmental cytokine milieu has important effects, including: preferential polarization of T cell immune response toward a Th1 phenotype, generation of mature DCs [50] from monocyte precursors and their survival [51]. Recently it has been suggested that reciprocal interaction between NKs and DCs might support the emergence of cytotoxic CD8 + T subsets from naïve T lymphocytes via an independent CD4 + T helper cell pathway [52].

Natural Killer T Cells

Natural killer T (NKT) cells represent an heterogeneous subset of thymus-derived T cells [53], which possess characteristics of both T and NK populations and exhibit a broad spectrum of phenotypic and functional complexity [54, 55]. To date, according to wide variety of surface markers detected on NKTs in humans and animals, three main subsets of these lymphoid cells have been identified [56].

The majority of NKTs express an invariant T cell receptor (TCR), consisting of an α-chain (Vα24-JαQ in humans) coupled with a β chain, and therefore this group of T clones is defined invariant NKTs [57,58]. These NKTs, by means of TCR, are able to recognize CD1d molecule, a ligand belonging to a group of glycoproteins, named CD1, which present a structure similar to MHC class I antigens. Therefore CD1 glycoproteins are defined non-classical MHC molecule [59]. CD1d is a marker shared by different cells, including antigen-presenting cells, B lymphocytes, myeloid cells and it has been also observed on cellular surface of some T subsets and healthy hepatocytes [60,61]. In a second population of NKTs, encounter of CD1d molecules is mediated by TCRs differing from TCRs exhibited by classical NKTs. A third subset of NKTs displays its effector function, via an independent CD1d recognition.

NKTs express further T lymphocyte receptors, such as either CD4 + or CD8 + or may be double negative as well as exhibit NK specific markers, including CD161 (NK1.1 in mice) and Ly-49 [62]. Following their activation NKTs rapidly release a broad pattern of cytokines, including IL-2, IL-4, TNF-α and IFN-γ, and display Fas, perforin, granzyme-mediated cytotoxic activity [63]. The pattern of cytokines secreted by NKTs is modulated by the type of receptor predominantly stimulated. High levels of IFN-γ, in absence of IL-4 production are secreted in response to predominant stimulation of NK cells.

Natural Killer T subsets elicit important and crucial regulatory effects on both innate and adaptive immune responses, stimulating in cross-talk the functions of NK, DC, B and T cells. Recently some researches suggested that a direct immunoregulatory loop exists between NKTs and T regulatory cells, which may reciprocally influence each other [67]. NKTs control T regulatory functions via IL-2-dependent mechanisms, whereas T regulatory cells may modulate NKTs activity via direct cell-interactions [68].

NKTs are detectable preferentially in the liver with a lower frequency in the spleen, thymus, bone marrow and lymph nodes and their role is essential in the immune responses against a number of pathogens, including viral infection [53].

T Cell Subsets

To date, in the heterogeneous population of T lymphocytes, usually involved in immune responses against viral infections, several T cell subsets have been characterized on the basis of their morphological and functional patterns [69].

According to the different expression of CD4 + and CD8 + homodimers on their cellular surface, T lymphocytes are classified into CD4 + T cells and CD8 + T cells, respectively. The following aspects of kinetics of T clones have been described in several studies, both during acute and chronic infections [70] :

1. models of CD8 + [13,71] and CD4 + T cell development [72,73], pathway of differentiation and phenotypic changes [74];
2. expression of specific markers on cellular membrane, patterns of cytokine production and functional properties against pathogens in the dynamic network of T cell subsets;

Within the same viral infection, wide and heterogeneous conditions of antigenic load levels, exposure and persistence seem to influence strongly phenotypes and functional features of CD4 + and CD8 + T clones [75].

In accordance to the state of activation/differentiation CD4 + and CD8 + T cells may be subdivided into naïve or antigen-experienced cells, both in humans and in mice [76,77]. Naïve T cell subsets have not yet encountered their cognate antigen, displayed by dendritic cells, whereas antigen-experienced cells have recognized their specific antigenic fragments, loaded on antigen-presenting cells, in the context of major histocompatibility complex (MHC) and have undergone to final stages of differentiation [78,79,80]. This pool includes either effector T clones, with the abilities to produce effector cytokines and to exhibit cytotoxic function, or memory T cells, with the property to rapidly respond to antigen rechallenge. The recognition of antigens by both naïve and experienced T cells is mediated by the T cell receptor (TCR) in an appropriate MHC setting. The engaging of TCR is a critical step in induction of T subset differentiation and fate.

A hallmark differentiating naïve from memory T cells is the regulation of T subsets homeostasis [81]. It has been suggested that the long-term survival of CD8 + [82,83] and CD4 + naïve-T [84,85] clones requires two critical exogenous signals: a continous contact with self-MHC antigens and IL-7 presence [86]. In addition, a minor role in supporting the longevity of CD8 + naïve T cells is played by IL-15 and, probably, by CD4 + T clones. On the other hand, memory T cell survival is not depending on self-MHC recognition. Indeed, it depends on periodic cell division and, in CD8 + T cells, is modulated by IL-15 [87,88,89]. Wide series of surface markers have been utilized to characterize clones of antigen-specific CD4 + and CD8 + T cells, according different stage of differentiation. The most important markers observed are represented by CD27, CD28, CD45RO, CD45RA, CD62L, CD127 and CCR7 in CD4 + subsets and CD5, CD25, CD27, CD28, CD45RO, CD45RA, CD62L, CD57, CD127 and CCR7 in CD8 + T subsets [90,91]. It has been shown in animals that at earlier steps of differentiation specific-T cells express the majority of surface markers, including CD45RO/CD45RA, CCR7, CD62L, CD7, CD28 and CD127, which are progressively lost at advanced stages [92,93]. At intermediate steps T cells expose CD45RO, CCR7 and CD27, whereas down-regulate CD28 and CD45RA [94,95]. At advanced stages specific-T clones exhibit CD45RO but are lacking in CD62L, CD7, CD28, CD127, CCR7 [75,96,97]. Memory T cells express CD45RA, CCR7 and CD127 [98,99]. Lanzavecchia [79] reported that the absence of CCR7 on cellular surface of specific-T cells would define sets of peripherical lymphocytes with effector activity (effector memory cells, T_{ET}), whereas the expression of CCR7 would characterize T clones, called central memory cells (T_{CM}), which are located within lymphoid organs and would function as precursors of effector cells. Heterogeneous combinations of surface cellular T markers have been used to establish a correlation between phenotype, function and differentiation. According to expression of CD45RA/CD45RO, CCR7 and CD127 or CD27 and CD28, both CD4 + and CD8 + have been subdivided respectively in four classes with different phenotypes and defined as [103] :

CD4 positive T cells
1. T-central memory cells (T_{CM}), expressing CD45RO, CCR7 and CD127 or CD27 and CD28,
2. T-effector memory cells (T_{EM}) expressing CD45RO, CD27 and low CD127, but lacking CCR7 or CD28,
3. T terminally differentiated cells (T_{ET}) expressing CD45RA, but with the loss of CD45RO and CD127 or CD27 and CD28,
4. T Effector cells (T_E) expressing CD45RO or CD27, but lacking CD45RA, CCR7 and CD127 or CD28 [75,355].

CD8 positive T cells
1. T-central memory cells (T_{CM}), expressing CD45RO, CCR7 and CD127 or CD27 and CD28,
2. T-effector memory cells (T_{EM}) expressing CD45RO, CD27 and low CD127, but lacking CCR7 or CD28,
3. T terminally differentiated cells (T_{ET}) expressing CD45RA, but with the loss of CD45RO and CD127 or CD27 and CD28,
4. T Effector cells (T_E) expressing CD45RO or CD27, but lacking CD45RA, CCR7 and CD127 or CD28 [356].

A further series of studies have suggested complex developmental models of both antigen-specific CD4 + and CD8 + T lymphocytes. Several Authors correlated their degrees of differentiation, according to the phenotype, to functional activities and to interleukins releasing abilities. Particularly, on the basis of IL-2 and IFN-γ production, they showed the existence of different patterns of surface markers, including CD45RA, CD62L, CCR7 and CD127 [100,101,102]. In both CD4 + and CD8 + T cell populations, the following different subsets have been characterized [103,104]:

1. at earlier step of differentiation CD T cells, defined T-central memory cells (TCM), express CD62L, CCR7 and CD127, lacking CD45RA. The majority of these T lymphocytes presents single-IL-2 releasing and proliferating abilities,
2. at intermediate stage of differentiation CD T clones, called T-effector memory cells (TEM), are devoid of CDRA45, CD62L, CCR7 and expose CD127 at low levels. This population includes both a subset of T cells, proliferating and secreting IL-2 and IFN-γ, and a subset of T lymphocytes non-proliferating and releasing IFN-γ,

3. at advanced step of differentiation T population, named T terminally differentiated cells (TET), expressing CD45RA but lacking CD62L, CCR7 and CD127, contain cells without proliferating and interleukins production properties,

4. at the terminal stage of differentiation pathway T cells, defined T Effector cells (E), are CD45RA, CD62L, CCR7, CD127 negative and lose proliferating and interleukins release abilites [105,106].

In the light of the latest reports several concepts, describing functions of T clones in viral infections, have been progressively revisited.

CD4 Positive T Cell Clones

In accordance with previous understanding, CD4 + T clones have been considered crucial to mount an effective adaptive immune response, providing an helper function to different immunitary cells.

Depending on interleukins production, T helper cells have been usually differentiated into Th1 and Th2 cells, the former secrete IL-2, TNF-β and interferon-γ, the latter IL-4, IL-5, IL-6 and IL-13 [107]. In the early phases of activation T helper-cell subsets may release a mixed pattern of cytochines, with heterogeneous combinations of IL-2, IL-4, IL-5 and interferon-γ. These cellular clones are defined Th0 [108]. Th1 and Th2 are actively involved in priming of naïve T cells, cross-regulating mutually growth and differentiation of virgin T lymphocytes, by means of their cytokines. As previously described, interleukin-12 and interferon-γ, released by dendritic cells (DCs) and macrophages, induce amplification of Th1 subsets, inhibiting Th2 clones, whereas IL-4, produced by basophils, mast-cells and CD4NK1.1T cells, favours the Th2 priming of naïve T lymphocytes and down-regulates Th1 response [109]. Nevertheless T helper cell stimulation does not cause, as inevitable effect, a polarization toward either Th1 or Th2 phenotype. T cell differentiation seems to be rather a stochastic event with no complete efficiency [110]. Depending on the probabilistic nature of T cell-DC contact, even in presence of strong polarizing factors, only a part of a specific responding T cells are induced to acquire effector activity and homing properties. In addition T lymphocytes, belonging to a specific clone, are subject to different levels of stimulation and undergo distinct thresholds of differentiation. The magnitude of stimulation of each specific T lymphocyte is dependent on the degree of TCR affinity for antigens and the ability to compete with other T subsets.

In the last years previously not identified functions have been attributed to CD4 + T lymphocytes, including lytic [111,112] and regulatory abilities. The existence of cytotoxic CD4 + T cells has been proved in animals and humans, and there is evidence that cytotoxic CD4 + T subsets are antigen experienced or memory cells, according to their phenotype. The pathway of differentiation of these cells is characterized by a progressive and sequential either down- or up-regulation of some cellular surface antigens, represented by the loss of CCR7, CD 27 and CD 28 and the gain of CD11a, CD57 and lytic granules with granzymes and perforin [112]. Following their phenotypic changes CD4 + T cytotoxic-cells should acquire lytic properties, although their role in human pathology is not yet completely understood. Nevertheless these cytotoxic CD4 + T clones have been observed in different pathological conditions, including viral disease such as HIV [113], CMV [114,115], EBV [116] HCV and HBV infections [117]. In addition in the population of CD4 + T cells, a subset of specialized T clones (called Treg or Th3) with regulatory properties and immunosuppressive function has been observed. T reg lymphocytes are characterized by the expression, on their surface, of several markers, including CD4, CD25 (receptor for IL-2), OX40, 4-1BB, CD62L and CTLA 4 (cytotoxic T lymphocyte-associated antigen 4). To date Treg cells have been subdivided into two classes: 1) natural T reg cells, which are generated in thymus, 2) T reg cells that emerge in periphery, following a complex course of induction. A hallmark of CD4-CD25 positive T cells is their ability to mantain host homeostasis and preserve self-tolerance in the periphery, by blocking the effector activities of CD4 +, CD8 + and NK cells. A tight regulation of Treg cells function is crucial to limit the magnitude of immune response, preventing autoimmune disorders and limiting tissue damage. On the other hand an excessive inhibition of activity of immunitary system, induced by Treg cells, may cause a failure in adequate control of tumors and infections promoting a state of immunosuppression [118]. Natural T reg cells, thymus-derived, via a cytokine-dependent self mantaining loop involving IL-2 and Transforming-Growth-Factor (TGF-β), stimulate conventional peripheral CD4 positive-CD25 negative lymphocytes to acquire a CD25 positive regulatory phenotype, exhibiting suppressive functions and secreting IL-10 and TGF-β [119,120]

CD8 Positive T Cell Clones

An effective CD8 + T cell virus-specific response plays a crucial role in immunological protection against patogens [121], with particular regard both to eradication of viral infection and to control of persistent and reactivating viruses, such as Cytomegalovirus (CMV) [122], Epstein-Barr virus (EBV) [123], Human Immunodeficiency virus (HIV) [124], Hepatitis B virus (HBV)[125] and hepatitis C virus (HCV) [126]. A coordinate and tightly regulated activity of CD4 + and CD8 + virus-specific T cells is a hallmark for an effective and persistently successful immune response [127,128]. Recent observations have also contributed to improve our understanding of the dynamics of CD8 + T-cell responses, during viral infection [129]. In an early phase of acute infection, naïve-specific CD8 + T cells, encountering their cognate viral antigens presented by professional cells, are primed, undergo a clonal expansion, with many rounds of antigen-independent division and acquire tissue-trafficking abilities and effector functions, exibiting cytotoxic activities and release of cytokines with anti viral properties, but are unable to proliferate and to self-renew [130,131]. Following the peak of immune response, once antigen clearance has been obtained, a large part of these effector virus-specific CD 8 T cell clones, called cytotoxic T cells (CTLs), experiences apoptosis, whereas a permanent reservoir of memory CD8 + T-cells is established. CD8 + T memory cells maintain the ability to divide and expand clonally, after cognate-antigen re-encounter. This function is crucial for an optimal immune response. Previous reports emphasized the role of CD4 + T cells in priming naïve-specific CD8 +T cells via interaction with a common antigen-presenting cells (APCs) [132], according to either a three-cell or two-cell model. The former model proposed that priming of CD8 + naïve T cells is induced by a direct interaction among CD4+ T cells, APCs and naïve CD8 + T subsets in a single step. These activated CD4+ T lymphocytes provide their helper functions, releasing several kinds of cytokines. In the latter model, in a first phase, CD4+ T cells interact with APCs and induce up-regulation of their costimulatory molecules. In a second step the primed-APCs engage in crosstalk with CD8 + T lymphocytes and induce their activation.

Nevertheless recent studies are showing that CD4 + T helper cells might be not required for induction of primary effective CD8 + T cell [130,133], on the contrary the presence of specific CD4 + T subsets seems to be crucial for development of a functional and protective CD8 + T cell memory [134,135]. In response to antigen rechallenge, CD8 + specific T memory clones, generated without CD4 + T cell help, show a decreased ability to proliferate and release cytokines [136] and a reduced competitive fitness in the network of different memory cells [137]. A report performed in mice, evaluating the need of CD4 + T cell help in the course of CTL induction, has suggested that a pivotal role is played by the precursor frequencies of cytotoxic-CD8 + T cells. In this model, when the frequencies of CTLs are high, an effective priming of CD8 + T clones is not depending on CD4 + T helper subsets activity [138]. Recently it has been also suggested that a key function of IL-2 is to confer to CD4 + T cells, during their priming, a long-lasting competitive survival advantage in the environment of lymphoid system [139].

The course, acute versus chronic, of a viral infection strongly influences development, differentiation pathway, functional state and phenotype of CD8 + T memory cells [70].

Using a mouse model of infection with two different strains of lymphocytic chorimeningitis virus (LCMV) (Armstrong and clone 13 strains, inducing respectively an acute versus a chronic infection), Wherry reported that CD 8 + T memory cells, emerging in animals with a self-limiting acute viral infection, exhibit three crucial properties [140]:

1. long-term antigen-independent persistence and progressive memory T cell differentiation and exhibition of high frequencies of several receptors, such as CD122, CD127, CD62L, CCR7 and antiapoptotic molecule, such as Bcl2,
2. spontaneous self-mantaining ability (called homeostatic proliferation), which controls the size of T cell clones, via strong response to IL-7 and IL-15,
3. efficient and rapid response after antigen rechallenge and IL-2 release.

On the other hand, in the absence of viral clearance a chronic infection develops and is characterized by:

1. poor antigen-independent-persistence, with impaired CD 8 T cell differentiation, low levels of CD122, CD127, CD62L, CCR7 and Bcl2,
2. no homeostatic proliferation and response to IL-7 and IL-15,
3. impaired immune response and IL-2 production, following the reinfection.

Therefore the critical features of CD8 + T memory cells in chronic infections are represented by the need of persistent exposure to antigen to survive, and the absence of homeostatic proliferation. If this functional dysregulation of CD8 + T memory cells represents a cause or an effect of chronic infections, it is not well-understood. Recent results are not completely consistent with this assumption [141]. The Authors have suggested that in chronic virus infection specific-antiviral CD8 + T cells present defective self-mantaining abilities and therefore lymphocyte naïve-antigen-specific CD8 + T cells are continuously primed and recruited to replace these antigen-experienced T subsets with short-lasting survival. This event leads to the generation of CD8 + T pools with marked phenotypic heterogeneity. A further study shown that virus-specific exhausted CD8 + T cells in mice persistently infected with LCMV present a long-lasting hyperexpression of the programmed death 1 (PD-1) molecule, a receptor with inhibitory activity of CD28 family. A transient exposure of PD-1 has been described in early effector CD8 + T cells in mice with an acute LCMV resolving infection, with generation of functional memory CD8 + T lymphocytes, PD-1 negative. Blockade of PD-1 in mice with LCMV chronic infection has restored the fitness of exhausted-CD8 + T subsets, also in the absence of CD4 + T helper cells [142], including the ability to proliferate, to release cytokines and to destroy infected cells.

In addition it has been observed that, in the pathway of immunitary cells differentiation following an infection, levels of receptors and markers expressed on cellular surface present wide fluctuations. In homeostatic proliferation, after the acute phase of an infection, when a specific-CD8 + T cell memory pool is established, IL-7 and its receptor CD127 have a key role. In the course of their differentiation pathway, naïve CD 8 + T subsets exhibit high levels of CD127 (CD127^{high}), but subsequently, after clonal expansion, mediated by antigen-encounter, become effector cells and down-regulate CD127 (CD127^{low} cells). After control of viral infection, CD127 is again up-regulated on CD8 + T cells acquiring a memory phenotype [143]. In recent studies performed in HIV-infected subjects, a continous viral replication has been related to a low expression of CD127 [144,145] and counts of CD8 positive-CD127^{low} T clones have been associated with clinical markers of disease progression, such as enhanced viral load and decreased frequencies of CD4 + T subsets [146]. On the other hand, viral inhibition elicits CD127^{high}-CD8 positive T cells [147,148], but the generation of a really effective pool of HIV-specific long-lived-CD127^{high}-CD8 positive T memory cells is observed, only if, after infection, an early antiretroviral-treatment (ART) is administered [149]. In chronically HIV-infected individuals, treated with ART, and even in chronic carriers with a long-term control of HIV-replication without treatment, frequencies of HIV-specific-CD127^{high}-CD8 positive T memory cells are low. T cells of these patients express predominantly an effector-function CD127^{low} phenotype. It has been suggested that in these subjects a constant viral replication induces a CD127^{low} CD8 positive T response to maintain low viremic levels, preventing the emergence of 127^{high}-CD8 T positive cell.

B Cells

Previous notions, concerning the role of B lymphocytes in immune responses, have been focused on their ability to drive the production of antibodies, by differentiating into plasma cells [150]. In recent years, the understanding of B-cell biology has been progressively enhanced. It is now accepted that B clones, in addition to provide humoral immunity, regulate the function of immune system via a multitude of ways. Although the priming of naïve T subsets is predominantly driven by DCs, B lymphocytes also act as antigen-presenting cells, activate CD4 + T subsets [151,152] and, like T cells, release a broad array of cytokines after antigen-stimulation [153]. These events depend on cytokine microenvironment in which B cells differentiate, following the interaction with their cognate antigen and cooperation with specific T helper cells. In the last years two different population of effector B clones (defined B effector 1 and B effector 2 cells), which produce distinct patterns of cytokines, including IL-2, IL-6, Il-10, TNF-α and IFN-γ, have been characterized [154]. Particularly naïve B clones, cultured in presence of antigen and Th1 subsets, differentiate into Be1 cells, which are able to release IFN-γ, upon restimulation. Naïve B lymphocytes, stimulated in vitro in association with Th2 and antigen, culminate into Be2 cells differentiation, with IL-4 secretion, following restimulation. Taken advantages from these results it has been suggested that a reciprocal regulation of polarized cytokine production by B and T populations exists and B clones cooperate actively with DCs, NK, NKT and T lymphocytes to generate an effective immune response and to control its development. In the starting phases of this process DCs, after recognition of their cognate antigen, migrate to the T cell zones of secondary lymphoid organs, to encounter specific-T helper cells [155]. Naïve B clones also may be detected transiently in the borders of T-cell/B-cell zones, where these B cells interact with antigen-primed specific-T helper subsets. The cooperation between B and T lymphocytes induces Ag-primed B populations to clonally expand and to generate both short-lived plasma cells, detectable in T zone of secondary lymphoid organs, and B clones which migrate to the follicles of B areas, orchestrating the generation of B cell memory [156,157,158]. Several molecules have been implicated in B-T cell interactions. The most important receptors, identified on membrane of B subsets and involved in B-T lymphocytes collaboration, are represented by CD40, CD11a/CD18 (or LFA-1), CD54 (or ICAM-1), CD80/86, OX40L, Fas, Ig-α/β, B7.h. These molecules interact with their cognate ligands on T cells, which are constituted by CD40L, CD54 (or ICAM-1), CD11a/CD18 (or LFA-1), CD28 (CTLA-4), OX40, Fas-L, CD3/CD4, ICOS [159]. Recent studies indicate also that B cells are crucial for the optimal generation of memory CD4 + T subsets, modulating the entity of primary CD4 + cell responses [160,161] as well as that invariant NKT cells possess a pivotal homeostatic role in development of humoral response, B cell function and memory [162]. The emergence of sustained proliferation and differentiation of human naïve B-cells needs three signals to be effectively established. The encounter of antigen with B cell receptor is considered the first step of the process and it is followed by a second stimulus, the T cell help [163]. Both signals, acting in concert, are necessary and sufficient events to stimulate initial proliferation of naïve B cells [164], but are unable to promote their expansion and differentiation. A third signal is provided by stimulation of specific TLRs, expressed on membrane surfaces of B lymphocytes, and it induces these cells to undergo clonal expansion, somatic mutations and class switching of immunoglobulin, with high affinity for specific-antigen [165]. The TLRs, including TLR2, TLR6, TLR7, TLR9 and TLR10, in humans have been detected only in memory cells and up-regulated on B cells, following B cell receptor engagement. It has been observed that TLRs triggering may be caused by different agonists, such as microbial products. B subset cooperation itself with different myeloid cell types modulate the quality of antibody response [166,167]. The final event of this process is characterized by the emergence of both long-lived plasma cells and memory B clones [168]. These data strongly suggest that important interactions and complex relationship exist between innate and adaptive immune responses.

Chapter III

Hepatitis B Virus Genome Organization

HBV is a small, non-cytopathic, hepatotropic DNA virus, member of the family of Hepadnaviridae [169,170]. It is composed of an envelope and a nucleocapsid containing both viral genoma, a partially double-stranded circular DNA molecule, only 3,2 kb in length, and hepatitis B core protein, the structural protein of nucleocapside (HBcAg). Viral genome contains four overlapping open reading frames [171]:

1. **S,** for the surface or envelope genes (pre-surface1 or pre-S1, pre-surface2 or pre-S2 and surface or S) encoding for the large, middle and small surface proteins, respectively,
2. **C,** for the core/precore genes, encoding both core protein (HBcAg) and precore protein, which undergoes post-translational modification to become hepatitis B e antigen (HBeAg),
3. **P,** for the polymerase reverse transcriptase, a multifunctional protein with a crucial role for viral replication,
4. **X,** for the hepatitis B x protein, with cellular and viral genes transactivator properties [172].

HBV genome organization is depicted in figure 1.

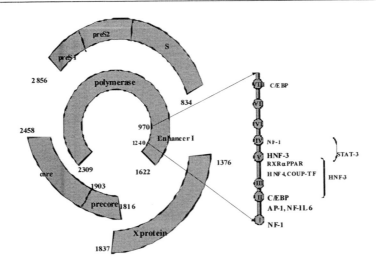

Figure 1. In this figure there are shown HBV genome organization and the most important binding sites for nuclear factor in HBV Enhancer I, such as HNF-3, HNF-4, AP-1, NF-IL 6 and STAT-3.

Chapter IV

Modulation of Specific Lymphocyte Subsets Response against HBV Antigens in Peripheral Blood and in Liver Tissue

It is now generally accepted that in HBV infection Thl-Th2 balance is a crucial factor in viral clearance or persistence, regulating the global host cellular and immune response.

A lot of immunodominant T and B cell epitopes, located on viral polymerase, envelope and nucleocapsid had been characterized in the last years, but dynamic sequence and kinetic of cellular and humoral immune response against such antigenic determinants in acute self-limited and chronic HBV infection are still poorly understood.

Hepatitis core (HBcAg) and e (HBeAg) antigens, representing two structural different forms of the viral nucleocapsid with a common region of 149 aa [173], had been proved to be very strong immunogens and play a key role in inducing T helper and T cytotoxic lymphocytes responses [174].

Activation of HBeAg/HBcAg specific CD4 + T cell clones appears to be essential in HBV clearance, promoting anti-HBe and anti-HBs antibody production and specific cytotoxic T lymphocytes proliferation and activity [175]. This component of immune response probably has a crucial role in viral eradication in patients with HBV resolving infection.

A lot of studies, examining immunitary cellular profile and cytokine pattern either in individuals with self-limited or persistent hepatitis have been performed respectively on peripheral blood mononuclear cells (PBMCs) and, concerning chronically infected subjects, on liver tissue specimens. A strong CD4 + nucleocapsid T cell-response with a prevalent Th1 cytockine release has been observed in T cells lines and clones isolated from PBMCs in subjects with acute self-limited hepatitis [176]. In HBV chronic carriers, both in HBeAg positive and HBeAg negative patients, clinical course of illness shows periodically acute exacerbations. These events are generally related to reactivated infection and are characterized by rapidly increasing viremia, before aminotransferases (ALT) flare develops [177]. These spontaneous exacerbations occur with different reported rates, with regard to series of patients examined, and may be understimated because of an asymptomatic course [178]. During these episodes histological changes, due to acute events, are associated with alterations induced by chronic damage. In a previous study, 22 HBeAg positive carriers were monitored for almost 26 months and their T cells responses against HBV recombinant core, HBeAg and envelope antigens were evaluated [179]. In these subjects it was observed that an initially increasing serum HBV-DNA and HBeAg concentration was followed by a strong nucleocapsid specific T-cell response with a flare in disease activity and subsequently a drop in HBV-DNA and HBeAg load. Some patients experimented HBeAg and serum HBV-DNA loss with anti-HBe seroconversion. Important hepatitis exacerbations may be observed also in carriers with precore-mutant HBV infection. In these patients viral genoma titres in serum progressively increase before flare occurrence, but HBeAg is persistently undetectable. The pivotal role of HBcAg specific CD4 + T cells in HBV clearance promotion has been recently underlined by Naoumov and coworkers. Eight Chinese patients with HBV chronic hepatitis were subjected to HLA-identical bone marrow transplantation (BMT), because of hematologic malignancy. Bone marrow (BM) donors had previously succesfully eradicated HBV. Surprisingly, irrespective of well-known low rate of HBV clearance reported in Chinese individuals, even under treatment conditions, six carriers resolved chronic infection and presented long-lasting anti-HBs seroconversion [180]. This result has been ascribed to adoptive transfer of CD45 R0+ HBcAg specific CD4 + T cells (with a memory phenotype), since this outcome did not occur in transplanted patients, when graft derived from subjects with a vaccine-induced immunity [181]. Among the nucleocapsid antigenic determinants known so far, core residues 18-27 and 141-151 are the dominant epitopes recognized in HLA I class restricted CTL responses, whereas core 1-20, 50-69 and 120-139 are reported to play a major role in HLA II class restricted T helper activity [182]. In this respect different HLA backgrounds may provide an effective and vigorous immunoregulation in antigen presentation [183].

A very important determinant in priming Th-cell phenotype is the structural form of nucleocapsid [184], whereas its particulate form (HBcAg) preferentially promotes a Thl response, its soluble form (HBeAg) elicits a Th2 cell subset [185]. Available data in transgenic mice, comparing immunogenicity of HBcAg and HBeAg, demonstrated that HBcAg is significantly stronger than HBeAg in Th cell activation and antibody production and it is both a T-cell dependent and a T-cell independent antigen [186].

A lower HBcAg dose (0.025 ng) compared to HBeAg dose (25 ug) is required to elicit a detectable antibody response in transgenic mice models. Consistent with Thl-like cells pattern HBcAg induces mainly an IgG2a and IgG2b antiHBc isotype profile, whereas HBeAg elicits an IgGl anti HBeAg production, according to a Th2-cells response.

Interesting observations show that low ribonucleic acid (RNA) amounts, containing one or more unmethylated dinucleotides (CpG) immunostimulating motifs, complexed with antigens, act as strong activators of both innate and specific response [187,188]. According to this issue there is evidence that ribonucleic acid, linked to arginin-rich C-terminal region of HbeAg, displays a crucial role in priming Thl immunity. Complete HBeAg particles are able to induce IL-12 and IFN-γ production by DCs and spleen cells respectively. Conversely HBeAg, devoid of nucleotide-binding sequences or mutants (144 or 149 aa long) HBeAg particles, lacking in region rich in RNA, and achieved by expression in recombinant bacteria or by deletion of the arginin-rich C-terminal region of HBeAg, elicits preferentially a Th2 immune response [189].

T-cell recognition site and MHC host genotype may also modulate the phenotype of HBcAg/HBeAg specific T-helper cells [190]. In B10.S (H2^S) mice strains HBeAg primed T-cells show a strong proliferative response and acquire the ability to produce IL-2 and IFN-y more efficiently than IL-4. On the other hand in B10.(H2^b) mice models, HBeAg elicits a weak proliferative response and a IL-4 production, prevailing over IL-2 and IFN-y release [191].

A more complex, subtle and dynamic cross-regulation between HBcAg/HBeAg specific T helper cells recognizing the same antigenic determinant in the context of dissimilar structural form of the antigen (HBeAg or HBeAg) and between HBeAg specific T helper cells, identifying different epitopes on the same antigen, seems to exist. In a favourable genetic background, such as B10.(H2^b) transgenic (Tg) mice, the secreted HBeAg appears very effective in inducing immune tolerance, probably by means of peripheral Fas-mediated apoptotic mechanisms [192].

Whereas HBeAg specific Th1 cells are deleted, HBeAg specific Th2 subsets survive and in addition may down-regulate specific HBeAg Th1 cell response by their antiinflammatory cytokines (such as IL-4 and IL-10) [193].

Intrahepatic immune response in patients with chronic HBV infection has been very difficult to study, depending on several factors, such as exiguity of hepatic specimens achieved by means of liver biopsy and difficulties in liver infiltrating immunitary cells isolation and characterization. Therefore understanding of immune response activity in hepatic compartment is still limited. Actually there are available few and heterogeneous reports with regard to immunoassay test used to identify lymphocyte-clones specifities, reactivities and cytokines pattern secretion [194,195]. Irrespective to these obstacles, nucleocapsid and envelope HBV specific T cell clones with different phenotypes and properties have been characterized [196]. In a previous issue a broad series of T cells subsets were isolated from liver-infiltrating lymphomononuclear cells and from PBMCs in 6 patients with HBsAg chronic hepatitis (2 HBeAg and HBV-DNA positive subjects, 3 HBeAb positive and HBV-DNA negative and 1 HBeAb and HBV-DNA positive) and tested according to their phenotype, specificity and surface markers. Irrespective of HBeAg presence/absence, the most intrahepatic CD4 + and CD8 + T cell lines expressed a Th0 like pattern, releasing IL-4, IL-5 and IFN-γ, whereas only 25% of these lymphocytes were Th1. In contrast the prevalent CD8 + T cells response observed in peripheral blood had a Th1 profile. In addition a greater proportion of liver-infiltrating T cells lines showed surface activation (HLA class II and CD69 molecules) and memory (CD45RO+) markers in comparison to low frequencies of circulating T lymphocytes with a memory phenotype. Surprisingly, although a low number of patients and T clones have been studied, lymphocyte lines isolated from liver did not express any antigen specificity, even for nucleocapsid epitopes, suggesting that in hepatic environment, during HBV chronic infection, the majority of T clones are not virus specific [197]. Therefore the liver milieu in these subjects might contribute to polarize intrahepatic T lymphocytes toward a Th2 phenotype. Recently HBeAg has been demonstrated to influence TLR signaling pathway. A reduced expression of TLR2 receptor has been observed on the surface of monocytes detectable in peripheral blood as well as of hepatocytes and Kuppfer cells obtained from liver of HBeAg positive patients with chronic hepatitis, with respect to both subjects with HBeAg negative chronic hepatitis and healthy humans. Down-regulation of TLR2 induced a decrease in TNF-α release.

In contrast, TLR2 and cytokine production were enhanced in HBeAg negative subjects in comparison to controls [198].

Fewer data about dynamic sequence of immune response against HBsAg are available. Although in chronic HBV carriers a production of antibodies anti-HBsAg (HBsAb) is undetectable with conventional immunoassays, in a considerable number of these patients low frequencies of HBsAbs may be proved with more sensitive tests [199]. Conversely, remarkable recent observations clearly demonstrate that, during the early period of an acute self limited hepatitis, infected patients are generally unable to develop a vigorous and strong specific HLA-class II restricted T cell response to HBV envelope determinants. Nevertheless, the late phases of infection in these subjects are characterized by HBsAg disappareance and progressive serum increasing amounts of anti-HBs antibodies, with subsequent development of protective immunity. The mechanisms causing these patterns of response are not understood. It is suggested that HBsAb production is mediated by a process of cooperation between HBV-envelope specific B cells, capturing and processing HBsAg epitopes and HBcAg specific T helper cells. In contrast HBsAg specific T helper lymphocytes might be functionally inactivated or deleted by rapidly increasing envelope antigens amounts. Anti-HBs antibodies possess a very effective function, because these are virus neutralizing antibodies [200,201].

Recently, a study performed in Trimera Mouse Model (a human/mouse radiation chimera, obtained by human PMBCs transplantation from chronic HBV patients or HBV immunized donors into irradiated and vaccinated with HBsAg Balb/c mice) has shown a vigorous HBsAg specific Th1 and B cells response in vivo in PBMCs isolated from subjects, who successfully eradicate HBV infection. The predominant HBsAb isotype profile in this model includes IgG1 and IgG2 antibodies subclasses.

On the other hand PBMCs obtained from HBV chronic patients did not displayed any detectable HBsAb production. These findings appear linked to a low HBsAg specific T helper lymphocytes frequencies rather than to a decreased HBsAg specific B cells number [202] and suggest an inadequate B cells stimulation by HBsAg specific T lymphocytes.

Among characterized surface epitopes, envelope 10-17, 109-123, 250-258, 260-269 and 335-343 are the most important HBV-specific CTL determinants, whereas envelope residues 10-19, 109-123 and 182-196 are recognized in HLA II restricted T helper response. In comparison to studies evaluating immune response against epitopes in HBc, HBs and HBe antigens, only few reports have described viral determinants on HBV polymerase. In acute self-limiting HBV hepatitis HBV polymerase has been shown to possess an high immunogenicity and to stimulate actively CD8 + T cell response. In the past, some antigenic determinants, such as 61-69, 445-463, 575-583, 773-782 and 803-811, have been described and have been shown to play a major role in HLA I restricted CTL responses [203]. A recent study has evaluated 66 HBV-infected patients, subdivided into 4 groups: group 1, 1 patient with acute self-limiting hepatitis who cleared HBsAgs and seroconverted spontaneously to HBeAb and HBsAb, group 2, 17 recovered subjects HBsAb, HBcAb positive, group 3, 14 chronically, not treated HBsAg positive patients, group 4, 34 persistently infected HBsAg positive subjects, treated with lamivudine. This study has allowed to identify 10 highly conserved and immunogenic CD4- MHC class II restricted epitopes, on HBV polymerase, located on the following aminoacid position: 96-111, 145-160, 385-400, 412-427, 420-435, 501-516, 618-633, 664-679, 694-709, 767-782 [204]. In accordance with data shown for CD8 + T cell responses against polymerase, an high frequency of patients with acute self-limiting B hepatitis elicit a strong immune response against at least one HBV polymerase peptide in comparison to a low percentage of subject with a persistent infection. It has been observed that also X-protein of HBV is immunogenic. Several sites within X protein has been demonstrated to be recognized by CD4 + T cells [205] including epitopes at position 11-25, 21-35, 31-45, 61-75, 71-85, 81-95, 91-105, 111-125, 120-135 [206]. The real impact of CD4 + T cell response, against X protein epitopes, remains to be understood.

Chapter V

Cytokines and Growth Factors Activities Induced by Viral Antigens during HBV Acute and Chronic Infection

In normal hepatic tissue a lot of effective and tightly regulated homeostatic mechanisms play a crucial role in cell growth and apoptosis regulation. Both cytokines and growth factors represent the mediators in the context of this dynamic network, controlling respectively inflammatory, apoptotic and immunitary responses or cell proliferation, differentiation, viability and normal liver physiology [207]. Therefore a precise and overall knowledge of cytokines and growth factors production, both in patients with acute and chronic HBV hepatitis, is mandatory [208]. The complex cooperation and interaction among these mediators constitute the main factors responsible for final outcome: viral clearance with recovery or persistence with a progressive disease, potentially evolving toward cirrhosis and hepatocellular carcinoma. During acute and chronic HBV hepatitis, immune response against viral antigens causes a liver damage, induced mainly by the intrahepatic inflammatory process, with variable patterns of severity.

A lot of studies have been performed to determine profile and cellular source of cytokines released in the course of HBV infection and have showed production and secretion of a large series of pro and anti-inflammatory cytochines such as IL-1, IL-2, IL-6, IL-8, IL-12, TNF-α, interferon-γ and IL-10 [209,210]. Moreover, interesting evidence is represented by HBV ability (according with several viral infections) to elicit specific and well-defined cytokine pattern secretion by host immunitary cells in response to its different proteins.

Particularly, as mentioned above, HBsAg has been demonstrated to induce mainly IL-2, interferon-γ and IL-10 [211], whereas HBcAg and HBeAg may stimulate preferentially a Th1 or Th2 cytokines like setting by T lymphocytes [212] and modulate IL-12 secretion by APCs.

In addition it has been proved that hepatocytes themselves may release several kinds of interleukins such as TNF-α [213] and IL-6 [214]. APCs function is performed in the liver preferentially by Kuppfer cells.

Among viral proteins responsible for cytokines induction, the HBx protein (HBx) appears to play a key role. It is currently accepted that HBx is essential for viral infectivity [215,216] and a likely cofactor involved in HBV carcinogenesis. HBx is a transcriptional activator with pleiotropic and different functions in host cells, depending on its intracellular compartmentalization and expression levels [217]. HBx may activate a lot of transcription factors, regulatory proteins normally located in an inactive state either in cell nucleus [218,219,220,221,222] or in cytoplasm [223,224,225]. These proteins, named Nuclear Factor of Transcription, binding specific cellular target genes, affect some important and specific cellular activities, such as development, differentiation, metamorphosis and physiology. Generally they are induced very quickly in response to environmental signals [226]. Binding sites of these nuclear factors, of IL-6 and of IL-8 are located both on cellular target gene promoters and on specific HBV regulatory sequences involved in viral transcription and replication, named Enhancers [227]. Up to date two Enhancers have been isolated in HBV genome: Enhancer I and II. The first partially overlaps to the X promoter and is included between X and S genes [228]. Enhancer I regulates X promoter and gene expression and it may be transactivated by HBx protein itself. Moreover Enhancer I includes at least five distinct binding regions, named 2C, GB, EP, E and NF-1 [229,230], where a lot of liver specific and ubiquitous transcription factors binding sites exist. Recent *in vitro* observations show that Enhancer I is responsive to AP-1 and Nuclear-Factor-IL6 (NF-IL6) [231], probably through a direct interaction between either AP-1 or NF-IL6 and specific E region sequences [232], harboring a c-FAP site [233]. Nuclear-Factor-IL6 is a component of the family of C/EBP transcription factors and its expression in hepatocytes is mainly enhanced in response to IL-6, IL-1 and TNF-α [234]. (Figure 2)

HBV Organization, Enhancer I and II and Nuclear Factors Binding Sites

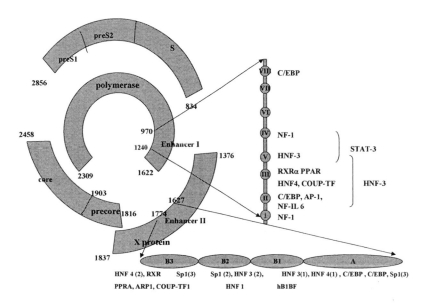

Figure 2. In this figure HBV genome organization and the most important binding sites for cellular nuclear factors in HBV Enhancer I and Enhancer II, such as HNF 1, HNF-3, HNF-4, C/EBP, RXRa-PPAR, AP-1, Sp1, COUP-TF1,NF-IL 6 and STAT-3, are shown.

On the other hand IL-6 may activate Enhancer I through an indirect mechanism: both IL-6 and Epithelial Growth Factor (EGF) are able to promote a tyrosine-phosphoprylation-mediated STAT-3 induction. Activated STAT-3 alone or in cooperation with Hepatocyte Nuclear Factor 3 (HNF-3) binds a specific HBV Enhancer I core sequence, leading to an overall stimulation of its function and viral gene expression [235]. IL-6 is a key cytokine, in the course of inflammatory processes, with pleiotropic functions such as cell proliferation and activation of acute-phase proteins in the liver. Increasing amounts of IL-6 are produced by hepatic and endothelial cells during acute and chronic HBV infection [236,237]. In addition it has been shown that HBV may control TNF-α production, another crucial cytokine involved in inflammatory responses. TNF-α secretion in HBV-infected liver may be demonstrated both in hepatocytes and in non-parenchimal cells. In HBV-transfected hepatocyte-derived cell lines, HBx protein has been showed to induce TNF-α synthesis through a transcriptionally up-regulated mechanism. Moreover the proximal region of TNF-α promoter includes several binding sites for nuclear factors, such as AP-1 and NF-κB. It is likely that HBx may up-regulate TNF-α production both by a direct or an indirect action. IL-8 promoter gene also may be transactivated through either NF-κB or C/EBP members interaction [238].

Chapter VI

Immune Response during HBV Acute and Chronic Infection

In accordance with several lines of evidence, it is now widely accepted that HBV itself is not cytopatic and that liver injury would be the result of immune response. Indeed, viral clearance, in patients with acute self-limited hepatitis, depends on a coordinate, vigorous and multispecific immune response, readily detectable in peripheral blood. In contrast it is weak or ineffective in subjects with chronic HBV infection [8].

The poor knowledge of HBV infection immunopathogenesis mainly depends on both an inadequate understanding of interaction between virus and host during incubation phase of infection and on absence of conventional experimental systems for its study. Since HBV is able to infect in vivo only humans and chimpanzees, whereas it is not infectious in vitro even for human hepatocytes, the relationship between HBV replication, liver injury and cellular immune response has been very difficult to investigate [8,239]. Nevertheless, in the last years, our understanding of viral biology and mechanisms involved in virus infection has been enhanced with the use of animal models infected with hepadnaviral homologues of HBV, and the introduction all of viral DNA sequences in genoma of transgenic mice. These mice replicate the virus at high rate in their hepatocytes and are immunologically tolerant to HBV, particularly with respect to T lymphocyte compartment [240]. This is an optimal model of persistent virus infection and its study has enhanced our understanding of viral biology and mechanisms involved in virus infection, although a lot of questions are not yet definied. In addition the characterization of HBV-circulating specific CD8 +

CTLs, isolated from patients who succesfully cleared the infection, and performed both in vitro by means of conventional chromium release assay and ex-vivo by HLA-A2/peptide tetramer staining [241,242], has allowed an accurate CD8 + T cells analysis, with regard to their phenotype, frequencies, specificity [243] and hierarchy of immune response. The combination of these immunologic tests may provide very precise determinations because prevents problems related to conventional chromium release assay use. Indeed the latter, requiring several cycles of PBMCs stimulation, may not detect the real amount of CD8 + T cells [203,244,245]. A possible limitation of the tetrameric technique depends on the small spectrum of epitopes till now identified and on the fact that the majority of antigenic determinants, which are generally used, have been recognized in a HLA-A2 restricted setting. These concerns suggest that real entity and magnitude of HBV-specific T cell responses might be understimated.

In the previous years a large series of researches in vitro, animals and humans have progressively contributed to develop the present knowledge of mechanisms involved in acute and chronic immune response to HBV. The key studies are reviewed in succession on the basis of their publication date in scientific literature from the early to the present reports.

First Studies Evaluating Immune Response against HBV from Eighties to Nineties Years of Twentieth Century

In 1982 a research evaluated, for the first time, the function of peripheral blood T lymphocytes, specific for epitopes of HBV core, showing that these cells could exhibit, in vitro, a cytotoxic activity against autologous hepatocytes, obtained from subjects with chronic hepatitis B virus infection. The results support the hypothesis that specific-T clones play a major role in the immunopathogenesis of HBV-induced hepatic injury [246]. Studies performed in transgenic mouse in the eighties have shown that HBV is not directly cytopathic for hepatocytes [247,248], suggesting that liver damage is rather related to the intensity of immune response. Adoptive transfer of HBsAg-specific HLA class I-restricted cytotoxic T cells in these animals has been proved to elicit a CTL-mediated necroinflammatory liver injury, with different degrees of severity, ranging from patterns of mild acute hepatitis to fulminant hepatitis, depending on several factors, including sex, amount of HBsAg in positive hepatocytes, size of liver cells expressing HBsAg, production of interleuchins and opportunity to manipulate the quantity and cytopathic activity of T lymphocytes [249,250,251]. Although at that time the knowledge of dynamics and functions of T lymphocytes was poor and, in the model of fulminant hepatitis proposed by Ando in 1993 [250], a large part of intrahepatic necroinflammatory infiltrate consisted of not antigen-specific T cells, recruited via an IFN-γ mediated mechanism, it has been assumed that HBV-specific-CTLs had a causative role in promoting both viral clearance and hepatic damage. In the next years further observations modified these assumptions, suggesting different conclusions: specific-CD8 + T cell response against virus would protect the liver from injury, rather than causing damage, both in animals and humans. Reports in transgenic mice secreting HBsAg demonstrated that several cytokines, released by HBsAg specific-CTLs as well as NK and NKT cells, such as IFN-γ [252,253], TNF-α and IL-2 [254,255] were able to mediate in vivo suppression of HBV replication and gene expression through non-cytolitic mechanisms. Indeed at a post-trascriptional level, they favour the degradation of intracytoplasmic HBV-RNA [256]. Similar results have been obtained in woodchucks [257] and ducks [258,259], infected with their species-related Hepadnaviruses. In the same years some studies were designed with the purpose to evaluate, also in humans, the immune response both during acute and chronic infection. These works were particularly focused on the role and kinetics of specific-CD8 + T lymphocytes, but a series of technical problems and ethical concerns complicated the implementation of a systematic research in this field [8,242,243]. The early studies, performed in acutely infected subjects, were confined to peripheral blood, without the support of sensible tecnique for *ex-vivo* longitudinal analysis of virus-specific-T clones [8]. This condition prevented for a long time an adequate characterization of dynamics of these cells in serum and hepatic environments and correlation with kinetics of immune response in subjects with persistent infection. The first researches identified immunodominant epitopes of hepatitis B virus specific cytotoxic-T lymphocytes in peripheral blood of patients with acute self-limited HBV-infection [174,244]. In particular some nucleocapsid epitopes have been isolated and resulted preferential targets for protective virus-specific T cells. Their activity, directed to these determinants, has been proved to play a crucial role for control and resolution of HBV infection. Subjects clearing the virus with success were able to mount a strong, multispecific, polyclonal and long-lasting CTL immune response against several viral antigens, readily detectable in serum. After recovery no biochemical signs of hepatic injury persisted in these individuals. In contrast analysis performed in patients with chronic hepatitis B shown that specific-T lymphocyte responses is weak or undetectable in serum and, when present, appears to be directed against single epitopes [260]. Nevertheless both biochemical and histological findings of liver damage could be observed in these subjects. At the site of hepatocellular injury CD4 + and CD8 + T clones, specific for HBcAg, but not for HBsAg, could be isolated and expanded from hepatic biopsies [261,262]. As reported previously in 1996 by Rehermann, irrespective of HBeAg presence/absence, patients with chronic B virus hepatitis, who showed a spontaneous or IFNa-related remission, mounted a multispecific-CTL response to viral determinants not differing from that detectable in patients clearing successfully HBV, with respect to CTL strenght, specificity and frequencies. In addition a specific CTL activity was observed also in subjects not resolving HBV infection: a prolonged in vitro peptide stimulation has been able to unmask CTL responses even in these patients [263]. In 1996 a further interesting study was performed in seventeen patients with a acute self-limiting hepatitis to evaluate viremia and HBV-specific T cell responses during the acute phase of infection and in the years following clinical resolution (for a period ranging from 2.2 to 13 years). This report provided the basis for the knowledge of long-lasting T responses directed to HBV, although, at that time, an accurate identification of the steps and the markers of T cell differentiation pathway was not available [264].

The study highlighted that:

1. circulating T clones with a fine specificity for nucleocapsid determinants were observed both in the early acute stage of infection and also years after recovery, following resolution of acute B virus infection,
2. peripheral blood T subsets CD45RO+, exhibiting the phenotype of recently activated cells, mediated long-lasting protection against virus,
3. approximately 50% of the patients were HBV-DNA positive by nested-PCR and memory T clones played a crucial role not only to prevent reinfection, but also to control virus reactivation.

The data from Jung and coworkers were consistent with these observations [265]. They tested virus specific HBc-elicited cytokine production and T cells proliferation in PBMCs isolated from patients with acute or chronic HBV hepatitis, by means of an ELISPOT assay, a more sensitive test than ELISA for cytokine measure in cell cultures. Specific CD4 + lymphocyte response with IFN-γ release, according to a HBcAg-induced Thl-like pattern, was detectable in supernatants obtained from T-cell cultures in both groups, with a low IL-4 production. The hallmark difference, emerging from this issue, between PBMCs isolated from patients with acute or chronic infection, is a more elevated number of cells secreting IFN-γ and consequently an higher IFN-γ amount, in the first group, providing a more efficacious antiviral response in these subjects.

Recent Advances in Knowledge of Immune Response against HBV

At the end of twentieth century progressive improvement in technology has supported the study *ex-vivo* of T lymphocytes kinetics during the course of viral infections [242,243]. Taking advantage of this opportunity several researches have evaluated the immune responses during the course of HBV infection. In 1999 a study performed in patients with HBV acute symptomatic hepatitis, utilized this technology to obtain *ex vivo* a direct phenotypic longitudinal analysis of circulating HBV-specific CD8 + T cells involved in the control of virus infection. This report described quantitatively the kinetics, magnitude, hierarchy and ability of clonal expansion of these circulating specific-T lymphocytes. These T clones reach the peak in frequency during the clinical phase of acute hepatitis [243], showing an activated phenotype with impaired and limited proliferative and cytotoxic abilities. A complete restoration of these responses has been detectable only after resolution of infection.

It is noteworthy, however that circulating CD8 + cells frequencies, specific for several immunodominant HBV epitopes, such as core 18-27, polymerase 575-583 and envelope 335-343, have never overcome about 1,3% of total CD8 + peripheral blood cells, even if isolated with tetramer staining assay. A study in 2000 evaluated immune response in woodchucks, infected with corresponding hepatitis virus, through the analysis of repeated serum and liver tissue samples [266]. After infection, the liver of woodchucks was quickly infiltrated by CD3 positive lymphocytes, reaching a substantial peak within 4 weeks in animals with resolving hepatitis. CD3 positive lymphocytes was associated with CD4 + and CD8 + T cell hepatic migration, 3-4 weeks after the start of infection. This event was followed by IFN-γ, TNF-α and IFN-α release. In liver tissue specimens, lymphomononuclear cells were widely scattered in the whole hepatic lobular structure, with apoptotic and regenerating hepatocytes foci. In contrast, woodchucks developing a woodchuck hepatitis virus (WHV) chronic carrier state, showed lower intrahepatic CD3 and CD 8 T cell frequencies, with lower levels of antiviral cytokines (such as IFN-γ and TNF-α) in comparison with the findings observed in animals with acute resolving infection. Liver histology was characterized by an inflammatory infiltrate, predominantly located in portal areas, spreading into hepatic lobule, with areas of piecemeal necrosis and structure subversion [267]. Therefore these data strongly confirm that CD4 + and CD8 + activation is crucial in HBV eradication, via both cytolytic and not cytolytic mechanisms.These findings had been suggested previously by Guidotti in transgenic mice models, and confirmed in 1999 in two HBV-infected chimpanzees, developing a self-limited hepatitis [268]. There is a dose resemblance between this animal model and human HBV infection [269]. Chimpanzees may be infected by HBV and their hepatocytes are able to produce cccDNA, the long lasting viral form, template for virus RNA synthesis [270]. Guidotti et al have showed that the not-cytopatic immune response in these animals also plays a key role in clearance from hepatocytes of cccDNA and its intermediate forms. This is a prerequisite condition for viral eradication, and it probably occurs at a post-transcriptional level. In accordance with the report by Ando also in chimpanzees with HBV infection hepatic injury is associated with a massive recruitment of antigen-aspecific CD8 + T lymphocytes.

In 2000 a further crucial study evaluated the dynamic course of HBV infection in a small group of patients, infected through a skin-piercing procedure (named autohemotherapy), and has allowed these subjects to be identified before the beginning of symptomatic phase of illness [271]. It has been possible therefore to observe, in these subjects, the clinical course of disease and examine HBV replication rates, serological profile of liver damage and kinetics of immune responses, studying mononuclear cells of peripheral blood, from the incubation phase to recovery. This research shows that, during incubation phase, HBV-DNA concentrations progressively increase and reach a peak approximately 8-10 weeks after infection onset. Afterwards a rapid decline in HBV-DNA amounts have been observed in association with normal transaminases (ALT) levels. Surprisingly a maximal reduction in circulating HBV-DNA was already detectable before the rise of ALT and the development of clinical phase in subjects proved to clear succesfully HBV thereafter. The only immunosuppressed patient in this study had not acute hepatitis, maintaining high HBV-DNA serum concentrations and moderate ALT levels.

During the incubation phase of infection an increasing rates of circulating NK cells have been detected both in acute and immunosuppressed subjects, then patients with self limited hepatitis mounted a strong CD4 + and CD8 + T cell mediated response, controlling virus replication and spreading. A study by Maini [272] in 2000 has evaluated the role of specific CD8 + T cells with regard to immunopathogenesis of HBV persistent infection. For the first time, frequencies, phenotypes, specificity and function both of circulating and liver infiltrating CD8 + T cells clones have been assessed in an organized and systematic fashion in HLA-A2 positive HBV carriers and tested by peptide-tetramer staining specific for the already reported epitopes (core 18-27, polymerase 575-583, envelope 335-343) [273]. These subjects were subdivided in two groups, according to biochemical, virological and histological parameters, including respectively HBeAg negative patients, with normal ALT levels, low viremia values and absence of liver infiammatory features and HBeAg positive individuals with ipertransaminasemia and high HBV-DNA titres and histologic signs of chronic hepatitis. The average number of circulating tetramer specific HBV CD8 + T cells, range from 17/50,000 in subjects with chronic active hepatitis to 54/50,000 CD8 + T lymphocytes in individuals without signs of liver disease. The lower frequencies of HBV specific CD8 + T cells in peripheral blood of the first group have been considered as a result of selective retention of these activated lymphocytes in the liver [272,274], where immune response against virus B occurs. Nevertheless, the hallmark emerging from this study, is that liver-infiltrating HBV-specific CD8 + T cells with effector function have been isolated both in patients with signs of liver damage and in subjects without active hepatitis. Surprisingly, analysis of intrahepatic core 18-27 CD8 + T cells on liver biopsies, examined with an immimostaining assay, dysplayed that absolute and total number of these specific T lymphocytes (showing an activated phenotype) are comparable in both groups, irrespective of biochemical, virological and histological parameters. In subjects without evidence of liver damage it has been observed a relatively low number of specific core 18-27 CD8 + T lymphocytes. restricted to hepatic lobules, where they are widely scattered among hepatocytes, without additional cells presence. In contrast, in subjects without an efficacious HBV control, liver lymphomononuclear cells infiltrate is located mainly in the portal areas, but involves also intralobular zones, resulting in necroinflammatory foci formation and normal liver tissue structure subversion. In these patients, specific CD8 + T cells, although present in elevated total number, are deep in a milieu of mixed and heterogeneous population of immunitary cells, including an high proportion of nonspecific inflammatory cells. The result, consistent with the previous studies proposed by Ando in 1993 and concerning a model of fulminant hepatitis in mice [250], is that the overall frequency of liver-infiltrating HBV-specific T lymphocytes is lower in individuals with signs of hepatic disease, in comparison with subjects without active hepatitis and low viral load [272]. Based on these findings it has been supposed that liver damage in these patients is related to nonspecific HBV inflammatory cells rather than to CTLs function. After recognition of HBV antigens, specific CD8 + T cells activate two different pathways to clear virus: inducing the necrosis of infected liver target cells or blocking viral replication at a post-transcriptional level, by means of antiviral cytokines release. These two distinct mechanisms probably coexist during immune response against HBV, but with well-distinguished effects and consequences. It is clearly established that during acute virus B hepatitis in animal models, and probably also in humans, almost the entire number of hepatocytes in liver is infected. Consequently a prevalent cytotoxic CD8 + T cells response with massive hepatic cytonecrosis might have deleterious effects for the host, resulting in a fatal hepatitis. Therefore it is actually thought that, in the majority of patients with acute resolving hepatitis, viral clearance occurs mainly without destruction of infected cells [8,254,255,272]. This condition probably is present even in chronic carriers, who successfully control HBV infection in Maini's study, as observed in hepatic histological specimens. In these individuals, as suggested by Rehermann several years ago [263], the immune response, although unable to clear HBV, maintains virus replication to low rate, preventing hepatic damage. In contrast subjects with signs of liver injury show a predominant cytonecrotic component of immune response, with formation of hepatic necrotic foci, rich in nonspecific inflammatory cells [272]. These findings seem to suggest that hepatic injury and viral control are independently determined events. Factors causing this massive recruitment of aspecific immunitary cells, as observed in liver infiltrates, cellular subtypes, as well as reasons for which this condition occurs only in some patients, are not well understood. Nevertheless it is currently accepted that, in the earlier step of this process, CTLs themselves, releasing several kinds of chemokines, attract, in the hepatic environment, antigen nonspecific lymphomononuclear and polymorphonuclear inflammatory cells [275]. They quickly exceed the CTLs proportion infiltrating the liver, and cause necroinflammatory foci constitution. It has been also reported that the recruitment of these cells may be partially blocked by inhibition of two well-defined chemokines: CXCL9 (chemokine ligand) and CXCL10. Production of these chemokines and their cognate receptor (CXCRS) is elicited by IFN-γ secretion in response to virus infection and is induced by macrophages, lymphocytes [276,277] and even by hepatocytes in cultures [278] or in vivo [279]. Surprisingly chemokines release abolition appears to reduce the severity of liver damage, but does not prevent recruitment of different proinflammatory cells, such as neutrophils [280]. These cells have been recently proved to produce a lot of mediators, such as interleukins (IFN-α, TNF-α, IL-1β, IL-6 and IL-12) and chemokines (CXCL1, CXCL8, CXCL9, CXCL10, CCL2, CCL3 and CCL4) [281,282]. It has been reported in a HBV transgenic mice model that PMNs are able to promote hepatic damage amplification, favouring nonspecific inflammatory cells migration in the liver. This event may be prevented by neutrophils depletion, resulting in CTLs function preservation and in decreased hepatic disease severity [280]. At this regard, several years ago Vierucci [283], studying children with HBV chronic hepatitis, showed an impaired neutrophil function, consisting mainly in increased oxidative metabolism and superoxide anion generation. In addition, both HBsAg positive sera and HBV components were able to promote a respiratory burst in resting neutrophils. The Author supposed a key role of neutrophils and free radicals in liver damage induction. At the moment therefore, as suggested by above mentioned reports, a key role in liver damage promotion appears to be played by recruitment of nonspecific inflammatory cells. It is noteworthy however that also human fulminant hepatitis B has been related to an imbalance in intrahepatic production of IL-12, IFN-γ and IL-10, as it has been already observed in murine models [284,285]. IL-12 induces Kuppfer cell proliferation, activated lymphocytes and macrophage migration in liver and promote an hepatic inflammatory response, prevailing in portal and central vein areas [286].

In 2002 a quantitative and qualitative analysis of circulating HBV-specific CD8 + T cells, HLA24-restricted, obtained from patients with acute self-limited or chronic HBV infection, has evaluated the differences in immune responses in these two groups of subjects [287], with results similar to data reported by Maini, in his previous study. A high frequency of peripheral blood HBV-specific CD8 + lymphocytes were detectable in patients with acute infection, with a progressive important decrease of these T cells, during the resolution phase. The large part of these cells have a CD28 ^{positive}/CD45RA ^{negative} memory phenotype in acute phase, whereas acquire a CD28^{negative} /CD45RA ^{negative} effector phenotype, following in vitro peptide stimulation. In the group of patients with a persistent HBV infection, no circulating HBV- specific CD8 + cells were detectable in all patients except in one, but following in vitro peptide stimulation, low levels of virus replication and absence of liver inflammation correlated with a detectable number of circulating HBV-specific CD8 + T cells in comparison to patients with high rates of HBV-DNA in serum and with hepatic inflammation, who exhibited no detectable frequencies of HBV-specific T lymphocytes. Although the Authors reported that in persistently HBV-infected patients analysis of CD28/CD45RA antigens could not be performed they suggested that T cells with a memory phenotype exist in individuals both with acute and chronic HBV hepatitis and probably the effector T cells detectable in serum could be generated by memory T cells.

In 2003 Thimme [288] suggested a causal association among CD8 + T lymphocytes response, viral eradication and hepatic injury, during HBV acute infection in chimpanzees. In this setting, control, CD4 + T cells-depleted and CD8 + T cells-depleted animals were utilized and kinetics of intrahepatic cytokines, lymphocytes, HBV-DNA and ALT were studied. Virtually all hepatocytes of animals were infected. This study showed that CD8 + T cells are required for control of HBV, whereas depletion of these lymphocytes prolonged the infection, preventing the onset of virus eradication and hepatic injury. Viral clearance and liver damage resulted to correlate with the presence of intrahepatic-CD8 + T cells. Depletion of CD4 + clones does not affect the outcome of acute HBV infection. Two antiviral functions related to CD8 + T cells were recognized to induce viral eradication, including an early noncytolitic activity, mediated by IFN-γ release and a cytolitic mechanism, destroying the residual infected hepatocytes.

In 2003 a further report showed, in serum of HBV chronically-infected subjects, that HBcAg specific T cells are able to exert an important role in viral suppressor functions and acute breaks are induced by the expansion of activated memory cells [289]. Tang, taking advantage from observations by Maini, studied the intrahepatic immune response in liver biopsies of patients with chronic HBV infection, focusing on analysis of immune effector cells (including CD8 + T lymphocytes, NK-cells and dendritic cells), effector molecules (such as granzyme and Fas-ligand), interleukins (TNF-α and IFN-γ) and immune mechanisms, involved in virus control and inflammatory hepatic damage [290]. Consistent with Maini's results, this report has shown that intralobular number of CD8 + T cells was lower in subjects with elevated levels of ALT, whereas intralobular-CD8 + T lymphocyte density was higher in HBeAg negative patients with low viremia. In addition higher values of transaminases were associated with increased number of cells granzyme-positive in portal areas and Fas-L positive within hepatic lobules, being Fas-L a marker identifying Kupffer and lymphoid cells. TNF-α and IFN-γ secreting cells were detectable infrequently in biopsies of these patients. Nevertheless, differing from Maini's report, this study has a potential limit, not evaluating the HBV-specificity of intralobular CD8 + T lymphocytes isolated from biopsies. In contrast, virus-specific immune responses in liver environment during acute self-limiting hepatitis have not been studied in humans for a long time, because of the difficult obtaining of hepatic samples for histological evaluation. Standard liver biopsy presents potential risk of complications [291] and this concern has delayed the knowledge of events which take place in the liver of these subjects and prevented the understanding of correlations between circulating and intrahepatic clones of virus-specific CD8 + T lymphocytes. On the basis of the important differences reported in magnitude of viral replication, pattern of liver damage and immune response chronic hepatitis B is now considered an heterogeneous disease. A longitudinal analysis, ex vivo and following stimulation in vitro, of CD8 + T cells exhibiting a specificity for structural and nonstructural epitopes on HBV proteins, has been performed in HLA-2 positive patients persistently infected with virus B, according to ALT values, viremia, presence or absence of HBeAg and hepatitis flare. A value of HBV-DNA equal to 10^7 copies/ml resulted to be crucial. Patients with persitent infection and viremia below this value had peripheral blood multispecific CD8 + T cell responses, mediated by core-, envelope and polymerase-T lymphocytes. It is now accepted that core 18-27 T subsets are responsible for virus B control. Patients with viremia above 10^7 copies/ml might occasionally present T pools specific for envelope and polymerase, but no circulating or intrahepatic core 18-27 CD8 + T cells resulted to be detectable. In this study no correlation between the pattern of circulating HBV-specific CD8 + T clones and entity of hepatic injury has been detected [292]. In 2006, for the first time, the use of fine-needle aspiration biopsy made possible and reliable [293] the contemporaneous characterization of the specific T cell immune response dynamics during human HBV infection, both in liver and peripheral blood, during and after acute viral infection [294]. This tecnique presents a good tolerability and may be performed several times [295]. Five HLA-2 positive adult-patients with acute hepatitis B virus have been enrolled in this study. Serum and liver samples have been obtained for a longitudinal analysis at first presentation and then soon after HBsAg clearance and, in 4 subjects, 30 and 90 days following HBsAb-seroconversion. This study has shown:

1. an higher ratio of total CD8 + and CD4 + T lymphocytes in liver in comparison to peripheral blood, showing a massive influx of CD8 + T cells in liver, with a correlation between intrahepatic compartmentalization of CD8 + clones and hepatic injury,
2. a predominant intrahepatic distribution of CD8 + T subsets specific for core 18-27 and envelope 183-191 of HBV versus serum (with values ranging from 1.2 to 21.7 folds), both during the whole course of infection and also after its resolution (with persistently high

percentages of total CD8 + T cells in the liver, soon after HBsAg
seroconversion and after 90 days), confirming strongly a key role of
these lymphocytes in HBV control,

3. a progressive decline of circulating- specific CD8 + T cells occurred,
    starting from the time of first presentation to that of HBsAg
    clearance.

4. higher frequencies of virus-specific T cells in liver with respect to
    blood, with most of these lymphocytes exhibiting an activated
    phenotype, (expression of HLA-DR at elevated levels) during the
    acute phase of infection,

5. a re-increasing percentage of activated-HBc 18-27 specific T cells in
    the liver of one patient, after 3 months post HBsAb seroconversion,
    suggesting reactivation of virus replication, followed by rapid re-
    emergence of epitope-specific CD8 + T clones, with a probable
    memory phenotype.

Potential limits in this study have been represented by the time of inclusion of
patients, who were enrolled only in the symptomatic phase of disease, therefore
lacking the incubation phase of infection, and by narrow spectrum of epitopes
available to characterize CD8 + T cells, by tetramer staining, probably
underestimating the real magnitude of specific-T lymphocyte responses. The
contribution of NK cells to the pathogenesis of HBV-liver mediated injury has
been re-evaluated recently [296]. The longitudinal study of patients with chronic
HBeAg negative B hepatitis, who experienced repeated hepatic flares, has shown
that large fluctuations of IL-8 and IFN-α in serum were detectable. A cross-
sectional analysis revealed that a strict temporal relation existed between hepatic
afflux of activated NK cells, release of these pro-inflammatory cytokines and
presence of active liver inflammation, these patterns being lacking both in
controls and healthy HBV carriers. It has been demonstrated that liver infiltrating
NK sets have acquired killing properties and have been able to induce hepatocyte
death through TRAIL ligand-receptor interactions.

In 2007 a study has evaluated the burden of different degrees of viral
replication and liver injury on the phenotypic and functional profile of CD4 + and
CD8 + HBV-specific T cells, according to recent rescheas on PD-1 molecule
function [297,298]. A longitudinal analysis in vivo of circulating-HBV-specific T
cell responses has been performed in chronically and acutely HLA-2 positive
HBV-infected patients, by using a wide panel of viral epitopes, covering the
whole viral sequence of genotype D [299]. Subjects with persistent virus infection

were HBeAb positive. This study confirmed that immune responses of circulating-HBV-specific T cell were vigorous in acute individuals, whereas were weak in subjects with chronic virus infection and, when observed, they were poor. In contrast IFN-γ production was observed both in acutely and in persistently infected patients. Viremia has been demonstrated to correlate inversely with frequencies and reactivity of specific CD4 + and CD8 + T clones, being high HBV-DNA levels associated with poor or undetectable lymphocyte responses.

In persistently infected patients the most CD8 + T cells detectable (0.02-0.08% of circulating CD8 + clones), specific for core 18-27, were CD127 (from 63 to 100%) and PD-1 (from 24 to 90%) positive, with high frequencies of these cells coexpressing either CD127 and CCR7 from 64 to 100%) or CD127 and PD-1 (from 55 to 98%). The phenotypic profile in acutely infected patients was characterized by an high percentage of PD-1 positive HBV-specific T lymphocytes (from 78 to 98%) with a weak expression of CD127 during the acute phase of illness, followed both by a reduction of PD-1 and an increase of CD127 after recovery. In contrast in subjects with chronic HBV patients CD8 + T cells presented a stable CD127 and PD-1 phenotype, suggesting that this pattern, induced by a high viral load, may be responsible of T lymphocytes dysfunction. The blockade of PD-1 and of its ligand PD-L1 was able to restore in vitro anti-viral immune response. Consistent with previous studies, evaluating mice inoculated with different lymphochoriomeningitis virus strains, it has been shown that in the early stage of acute viral infection low frequencies of virus specific-CD8 + T cells, expressing CD 127 (interleukin-7 receptor alpha chain), were detectable. In the following memory phase an high number of CD8 + T lymphocytes were CD127 positive [300]. It has been proposed that CD127 is an early marker identifying CD8 + T subsets committed to acquire phenotypic and functional characteristics of memory cells [301]. In the course of viral infection development of specific-CD8 + T lymphocyte populations expressing CD127 on cellular surface would depend on low viral load and adequate CD4 + T cell-help [302,303], whereas elevated and persistent levels of antigen would inhibit the emergence of CD127 positive subsets [304]. On the basis of these data Boettler studied longitudinally peripheral blood mononuclear cells from six HLA-2 patients with acute resolving B hepatitis. An accurate analysis of kinetics of different T cellular surface markers was provided by this report, in relation to the stage of infection, viral load, disease pathogenesis, functional and phenotypical T cell features. During the early step of acute hepatitis specific T cells did not express CD127 and lymph node homing receptor CCR7, whereas were CD38 positive. In the recovery phase the emergence of CD127 and CCR7 was associated with the down-regulation of CD38 and PD-1, the decrease of alanine aminotransferase and clearance of HBV. The Authors suggested that CD127 negative-CD8 + T clones presented phenotypic and functional characteristics of effector memory cells with limited proliferative abilities, whereas CD127 positive-CD8 + T lymphocytes exhibited a pattern corresponding to that of central memory cells, reported above, with the capacity to expand vigorously, but weak IFN-γ production [305]. According to results available, one might speculate that, in early phase of HBV infection, the emergence of central T memory cells is a crucial event to determine the outcome of infection, contributing to create a reservoir of cells with high proliferative abilities and self-renewal properties. In HBV chronic patients, factors affecting the differentiation pathway of these CD8 + subsets, such as hyperexpression of PD-1/PD-L1 complex [306,307,308], may block the maturation of CD127-negative-CD8 + T subsets, preventing these cells to express CD127 and to acquire a self-mantaining functional phenotype. This event might cause a depletion or unsuccessful emergence of a pool of central memory cells, a probably necessary condition to establish an effective, protective and long-lasting anti-HBV immune response.

Gehring has recently evaluated in 2007 the interplay between virus-specific CD8 + T cells and HLA-2 positive human hepatocytes either HBV-infected or not infected, to examine the impact of fluctuations in viral burden on CD8 + T lymphocyte immune response mediated by liver cells [309]. Several crucial aspects emerged from this study:

1. hepatocytes appeared to exhibit viral determinants to specific-T cells with poor efficiency, in comparison to professional APCs, although the mechanisms causing this default were poorly understood,
2. antigenic viral load modulated the type of antiviral CD8 + T cell function. Particularly, high rates of viral replication and antigens induced hepatocytes to stimulate a strong cytokine secretion by specific CD8 + T lymphocytes, whereas low antigenic load elicited preferentially degranulation of T subsets, with release of perforine and granzime, causing hepatocytes killing.

A study performed in HBV transgenic mouse, following adoptive transfer of HBeAg specific T clones, was consistent with this hypotesis suggesting that these cells might exhibit an oscillatory activity, ranging from non-cytolityc to cytolytic functions. These two opposite aspects of specific-CD8 + T immune-responses seem to depend on fluctuation of antigenic viral load expressed on hepatocellular surface at different time [310].

Therefore it has been suggested that the pathogenesis of HBV infection might be influenced by levels of viral load [8]. The peak in HBV replication, occurring during either the early phase of acute infection or following viral reactivation in the course of chronic B virus hepatitis, might induce the production of cytokines by specific CD8 + T cells, leading to viral control by means of non-cytolitic activities, but with subsequent recruitment of non-specific inflammatory cells [309]. On the other hand low levels of viremia might stimulate CD8 + T lymphocyte degranulation, promoting hepatocyte damage, without HBV clearance.

Chapter VII

Antiviral Treatments and Immune Response in HBV Infection

On the basis of assumption that CD4 + and CD8 + T cell hyporesponsiveness plays a crucial role in the establishment of HBV persistent infection and that, in patients with chronic B hepatitis, this condition is potentially reversible, therapeutic strategies have been developed to increase these defective immune responses and to restore T lymphocyte reactivity. In the last years, a lot of antiviral drugs have been licensed for clinical practice [311]. They quickly and strongly inhibit HBV-DNA synthesis in subjects with chronic HBV infection [312]. Unfortunately it is not understood whether the deficit reported in immune system activity is the cause or the effect of HBV infection.

The introduction of antiviral compounds, as possible alternative to interferon treatment, has provided further interesting data about immuno-pathogenesis of HBV chronic infection. Ferrari et al performed two clinical studies in patients with HBeAg positive chronic hepatitis, evaluating CD4 + T helper and CD8 + CTL cell responses before and during lamivudine therapy [313,314]. Twelve patients with chronic HBeAg positive hepatitis were enrolled in the first study to receive 12 months of lamivudine treatment (100 mg once a day), with 6 months of follow-up before and after therapy. Antiviral drug induced a dramatic drop in serum HBV-DNA load, temporally followed by an increased nucleocapsid antigens CD4 + T cell response. Particularly, circulating HBeAg specific T helper cells frequencies during antiviral therapy, reached levels comparable to rates observed in patients with acute-self limited hepatitis (from 1 specific positive T cells in 300,000 total T cells before treatment, to >1: 50,000 total T cells). The enhanced nucleocapsid T cell response was already detectable 1-2 weeks after the beginning of lamivudine. Furthermore, the effect of this antiviral drug in CTL response has been assessed in a group of 6 HBeAg positive chronic carries. These subjects were monitorized for 6 months before therapy and then treated with lamivudine (100 mg once a day for 12 months). There was also a follow-up period (6 months) after drug discharge. Particularly, behavior and frequencies of CTLs responses were studied, evaluating a broad panel of HLA-A2 restricted epitopes by means of both HLA-A2 peptide tetramer staining and chromium release assay. Following a rapid and strong decrease in HBV-DNA levels, induced by antiviral treatment, Ferrari and coworkers observed the appearance of wide and multispecific CTL reactivities against multiple HBV epitopes, not measurable before lamivudine administration. Nevertheless specific CTLs frequencies observed in patients during antiviral therapy were comparable to those detectable in subjects with acute self-limited hepatitis, only during the starting and ending phases of infection. CTLs proportions in chronic HBV treated carriers never overlap maximal peak levels observed in patients, who successfully eradicated virus. An earlier CTLs appearance was remarked in subjects under lamivudine therapy, when CD8 + T lymphocyte response was studied by means of tetramer staining in comparison to chromium release assay. The first immunotest provided a characterization of total circulating HBV specific CD8 + T cells, but did not measure their functional state. It has been suggested that a part of these lymphocytes, although really present, was unable to perform its cytotoxic function, therefore it was not detectable by chromium relase assay. A further study in 2003 [315], evaluating the long-term effect of lamivudine treatment in patients with HBeAg positive chronic hepatitis, showed that anti-viral functions of circulating-HBV-specific CD4 + and CD8 + T lymphocytes were only transiently restored under therapy with this nucleotide-analogue. Particularly the T cells responses were characterized by a bi-phasic course, an increase in T cell frequencies and reactivities, detected in the starting phases of therapy, was followed by a permanent decrease of T lymphocyte responses beginning from 5th-6th month of lamivudine administration. The origin of reconstituted circulating-virus-specific T cells, detectable in peripheral blood of HBV-infected patients treated with lamivudine, has been investigated in two subjects with B chronic hepatitis [316] and attributed to precursor T lymphocytes within secondary lymphoid organs, such as portal lymph nodes. These T subsets presented the ability to expand in vitro, following the stimulation with specific antigen and to release a wide pattern of cytokines. The hypothesis that liver participates in this process, releasing terminally differentiated T lymphocytes in blood, has not been confirmed in this report. Expanding his previous observations, Tang studied forty chronic HBeAg positive patients, randomized to receive either lamivudine or IFN-α therapy and analysed the number of pre-treatment intrahepatic CD8 + T-cells, HBcAg expression and response to antiviral therapy, showing, in liver biopsies, an higher pre-treatment values of CD8 + T lymphocytes and a slightly lower nuclear HBcAg expression in responders in comparison to non-responders. A correlation was detected between number of CD8 + T lymphocytes and hepatocytes expressing HBcAg in cytoplasm. In addition he observed a significative reduction of nuclear and cytoplasmic expression of HBcAg in hepatocytes as many as in number of CD8 + T cells, during the course of therapy, only in responding subjects, irrespective of treatment administred. Unfortunately it has not been determined whether CD8 + T cells were HBV-specific [317]. In a further report Tang examined longitudinal intrahepatic CD8 + T cell response in 20 HBeAg positive subjects, treated with pegylated-α-interferon for 52 weeks, using the FNAB-technique and shown that a significant enhancement of total-CD8 + T cells was detectable in responders in comparison to non-responders. An effective immune response was characterized by the following aspects: an increase of CD8 + granzyme and IFN-γ positive cells, no change in CD4 + T cells and reduction in CD56 positive NK cells. Patients not responding to this therapy exhibited an enhancement in intrahepatic NK cells, without variations in the number of CD4 + and CD8 + T lymphocytes [318]. The peptide YMDDVVLGA, corresponding to aminoacid residues 551-559 of HBV polymerase, contains tyrosine-methionine-aspartate-aspartate (YMDD) motif [203]. The correlation between anti YMDD motif CTL activity and the efficacy of lamivudine treatment has been investigated in 14 HLA2 positive patients with chronic hepatitis B [319]. Complete and sustained responders presented stronger CTL responses toward both YMDD and its variants, including YVDD and YIDD, in comparison to non responders. In addition sustained responders exhibited an increasing frequencies of YMDD/YVDD/YIDD specific CTLs with effective functions with respect to non-responders. Recently a study in subjects with chronic hepatitis B has evaluated the impact of adefovir treatment on some aspects of antiviral immune responses. Several dysfunctions have been observed both in myeloid (mDCs) and plasmacytoid (pDCs) dendritic cells in patients with chronic HBV infection in comparison to healthy volunteers [339]. Taking advantage from these results, number, phenotype and activity of these cellular populations have been analysed sequentially in peripheral blood of a group of individuals with chronic hepatitis B, during the course of treatment with adefovir. Six months of therapy induced a decrease in viremia equal to about 5 $\log_{10}$, normalization of ALT and a significant enhancement in frequencies of mDCs, which exhibited also improved abilities in secreting IL-12 and TNF-α. On the other hand no changes in pDCs function, reactivity and phenotype were detected [320]. Similarly the same group of Authors has shown that inhibition of viral replication after three months of adefovir administration was able to induce a decrease in frequencies of circulating-T regulatory cells, with normalization of ALT and a decrease in viremia in patients with persistent HBV infection. The reduction of serum T-regulatory cells was associated with an increase in proliferation and frequencies of cells releasing IFN-γ, following stimulation with HBcAg [321]. Recent reports have shown that peripheral serum monocytes of subjects with chronic B hepatitis present a down-regulation of the TLR2 receptor, its expression being improved by an effective lamivudine treatment [322].

Chapter VIII

Possible Mechanisms and Events Involved in Immune Response Dysfunctions in HBV Chronic Infection

Potential quantitative and qualitative dysfunctions, affecting the efficacy of innate or adaptive immune response during viral infection, may contribute to cause its persistence [323]. A noncytopathic virus, such as HBV, may cause the emergence of a chronic infection, overcoming, not inducing or evading host immune response, by means of different mechanisms [324].

A lot of possibilities have been described:

1. infection of immunologically privileged sites,
2. emergence of epitope escape virus mutants,
3. defective antigenic viral epitopes processing by APCs,
4. imbalance in cytokines production or release (for details, see paragraph entitled: CYTOKINES AND GROWTH FACTORS ACTIVITIES INDUCED BY VIRAL ANTIGENS DURING HBV ACUTE AND CHRONIC INFECTION)
5. negative central selection or clonal peripheral deletion of virus specific T-cells,

6. peripheral lymphocytic anergy of virus-specific T cells, which
    escape clonal deletion, but exhibit a poor ability to perform an
    effective immune response.

Infection of Immune Privileged Sites

Viral immune escape may result by sequestration of viruses in sites
inaccessible to effector cells of immune system, preventing an efficacious and
protective immune response [325]. Replicative forms of HBV have been detected
in several organs throughout the body, including mesenteric lymph nodes, spleen,
kidney, pancreas, testis, ovary, adrenal and thyroid glands [7,326]. Microvascular
barriers, lacking in the hepatic microenvironment, are generally present in the
majority of different tissues and may preclude the access to antigen specific-
cytotoxic T lymphocytes, preventing their antiviral activity at the sites of
infection. This situation has been described to occur in pancreas and kidney
[327]. In HBV transgenic mice, expressing viral antigens in liver and kidney,
specific T lymphocytes with cytotoxic activity are able to induce hepatitis, but not
nephritis. Therefore several organs are preserved by immune-mediated damage,
but may constitute a reservoir of virus, which may continuously reinfect the liver
and promote the establishment of viral persistence.

Emergence of Epitope Escape Viral Mutants

A further mechanism by which virus may evade immune response is
represented by generation of epitope mutations with loss of antigenicity.
Naturally or treatment-induced changes in HBV genome may elicit virus variants
with reduced immunogenicity [328,329,330]. A selective immunological pressure
on the virus may be exerted by functionally active CD8 + antigen-specific T cells
themselves, favouring the development of escaping viral variants [331]. In
particular down-regulation of MHC class I molecule [332] as many as mutations
emerging in viral determinants, recognized by TCR of specific-CD4 + and CD8 +
T cells, may prevent T lymphocyte encounter with its cognate antigen or
antagonize it, therefore abrogating the crucial starting phases of adaptive immune
response [262,333]. Changes involving pre-core/core genes cause the
development of HBV populations unable to secrete HBeAg, a critical target for

immune response, therefore promoting virus persistence. In addition mutational inactivation of B cell epitopes have been described in HBV persistently infected humans, precluding recognition by antibodies [333,334,335,336]. A series of researches have isolated HBV strains, bearing changes in the envelope gene. These mutations prevent expression of detectable HBsAg, resulting in the emergence of antibodies against HBsAg, despite the persistence of HBV infection [337,338].

Dendritic Cell Dysfunction

Few but remarkable observations suggest a critical role of DCs dysfunction as further cause of defective immune response in patients with HBV chronic hepatitis. Peripheral blood DCs, isolated from subjects with HBV persistent infection and cultured in vitro, showed an immature phenotype and an impaired ability to present HBV antigens to specific T cells, in comparison to DCs from healthy donors [339]. This result apparently disagrees with data obtained by Rossol and collegues. They studied the immunoregulatory role of IL-12 in 72 subjects, chronically infected by HBV. These carriers were reported to have higher serum basal amounts of IL-12 and IL-12p40 with respect to controls. Furthermore HBcAg-specific immune response was evaluated during an IFN-a course of therapy in 33 of 72 patients with HBeAg positive chronic hepatitis. The treatment induced in 10 of 33 subjects a sustained HBV-DNA disappareance and seroconversion to anti-HBe, with considerable adjunctive enhanced production of IL-12 and Thl-like cytokines. Moreover, a substantial increase in HBcAg-specific T cell response, in dose association with hepatocytes necrosis, was detectable during IFN-a therapy in 23 patients (8 responders and 15 non-responders), who experimented a remarkable hepatic cytonecrosis. Surprisingly, ALT flare advanced IL-12 peak, whereas anti-HBe seroconversion developed before or in concomitance with IL-12 maximal serum levels [340]. This study provides further evidence on key role of IL-12 and its cellular sources (DCs) in promoting an effective response against HBV. In addition it confirms the central immunoregulatory role of HBcAg-specific T cells response. According to observation reporting an impaired DCs function during HBV chronic infection, present studies are pointing to develop therapeutic immunization strategies to break HBV T-lymphocytes tolerance. Transgenic mice were infused with cytokine-activated bone marrow derived DCs. The procedures restored DCs function and consequently improved HBsAg specific CTLs function. These cells were detectable also in not treated animals, but they were devoid of effector activities. On the other hand, different mechanisms might impair or destroy DCs, favouring CTLs unresponsiveness. It has been suggested that APCs, processing viral antigens, might be themselves the target of CTLs action. Alternatively, CTLs inadequate stimulation might result in CTLs unresponsiveness. Systemic administration of an antiCD40mAb (monoclonal antibodies), endowed with agonistic properties, in an HBV transgenic mice model has been able to induce hepatic APCs activation and to promote their complete maturation. This event results both in a noncytopathic block of HBV replication, linked to direct APCs or different immunitary cells (NK and T lymphocytes) cytokines production and in stimulation of specific CTLs function. Therefore activation of this process may have a very useful role in HBV control [341].

T Lymphocyte Dysfunction

Recent studies have shown that different steps of the normal CD4 + and CD8 + T lymphocyte responses, detectable during an acute viral infection, become rapidly impaired after the establishment of a persistent infection [342,343]. This event, promoted by exposure to high antigenic viral load and enhanced levels of viral replication, induces a profound impact in CD8 + T cell activities and properties, causing: 1) an alteration of normal hierarchical immunodominance of CD8 + T subset responses, 2) a modification of tissue distribution of virus-specific CD8 + T lymphocytes, 3) a hierarchical loss of effector and functional responses of CD8 + populations [344,345,346]. Distinct mechanisms may be involved in CD8 + T cells overall imbalance and may differ even as a consequence of age in which HBV infection is acquired. Viral transplacental transmission in children born from HBeAg chronically infected mothers is able to elicit HBV persistence, probably by means of predominant HBV-specific naive T-cells thymic clonal deletion [8,345]. In adults carriers antigen and HBV-DNA overload may result in T lymphocytes tolerance by coexisting and cooperating mechanisms, such as exhaustion, apoptosis, clonal anergy and deletion [343,346]. A study has characterized the abilities and effector functions impairments of HBV-antigen-specific CD8 + T clones, surviving in patients with chronic HBV infections and high levels of antigenemia. A small population of CD8 + T cells with altered tetramer binding properties and a specificity focused on envelope antigen was detected and demonstrated to escape inactivation [346]. A recent study in LCMV-infected mice has analysed CD4 + T subset activities following an acute or chronic course of infection. CD4 + T clone responses were initially similar in both groups of animals. In mice developing a persistent infection an early CD4 + T cell inactivation was induced, with a hierarchical loss of functions [343]. At first, CD4 + T subsets become unable to release IL-2 and TNF-α, then to generate memory responses. Loss of CD4 + T cell function was strongly associated with CD8 + T lymphocyte exhaustion, suggesting that the cooperation between CD4 + and CD8 + T cells is essential to establish an appropriate and effective immune responses. Nevertheless a small fraction of CD4 + T lymphocytes survived inactivation and persisted despite chronic infection [343].

A further study has evaluated the kinetic, vigor and quality of responses of circulating-CD4 + and CD8 + T cells in 16 HLA-2 positive patients, with HCV acute hepatitis to examine the separate contribution of these T subsets in viral control and clearance [347]. These subjects were enrolled at the moment of clinical onset of symptoms. In all subjects circulating-CD8 + T subsets presented impaired functions, irrespective of infection outcome. In contrast, at this step, patients destined to control virus showed serum virus-specific CD4 + T helper clones with a polarization toward a type 1 phenotype and with strong activity and this event was followed by progressive emergence of central memory CD8 + T cells CD127 and CCR7 positive. In contrast subjects with non-resolving infection, CD4 + T subsets exhibited, in the early stage of infection, narrow, weak and poor responses with long-term persitsence of virus-specific defective CD8 + T populations, with CD127 and CCR7 negative phenotype [347].

These results confirm a previous report by Zajac and coworkers, who have demonstrated that mice infection with a particular LCMV strain (lymphocytic choriomeningitis virus) induced a CTLs and CD4 + T helper cells dysfunction, persisting for a long time, even after an efficacious virus control by immune response has been obtained [348].

In summary the hallmark, emerging from these studies, is that HBV-DNA levels and antigenic viral load are key and critical factors in promoting and mantaining T-cells hyporesponsiveness in patients with chronic HBV infection. Drop in viremia, induced by treatment with nucleo(s)tide analogues, is able to enhance CD4 + and CD8 + T-cell responsiveness. Unfortunately, this reconstitution is not enough to clear the virus in chronic carriers. A lot of causes, responsible for inadequate recovery in CD4 + and CD8 + T cell reactivity, under antiviral treatment are possible; covalently closed circular DNA (cccDNA) long half-life favours viral persistence [349] and high mutation rates in HBV genoma, arising as result of error proneness of polymerase (reverse transcriptase is devoid of a proofreading function), may promote appearance of nucleo(s)tide analogues resistant HBV strains with strong replication capacity. In addition duration of exposure to antigens is probably a critical parameter, affecting T cell responsiveness. CTLs prolonged antigenic stimulation, as observed in chronic infections, such as during HBV non-resolving hepatitis, in association with an impaired and inadequate CD4 + T helper cooperation, has deleterious effects on CTLs functional activities [342,346,347].

T Regulatory Cell Function in HBV Infection

It has been suggested that also CD4-CD25 + T regulatory cells might modulate the magnitude of CD8 + T cell-mediated immune response, during HBV infection. Stoop reported an increased proportion of peripheral blood T reg subsets in subjects with HBV chronic infection, causing the inhibition of HBcAg-specific T cell proliferation and IFN-γ production, in a dose-dependent manner [350]. In HBeAg positive subjects higher number of T reg cells were observed in comparison with HBeAg negative patients, whereas no relation was detectable among viral burden, hepatic injury and percentage of serum T reg lymphocytes. In contrast, no difference in frequencies of T reg subsets were described in different groups of subjects with HBV chronic or resolved were reported by further studies [351,352]. Nevertheless these reports demonstrated that serum CD4-CD25 positive lymphocytes suppressed ex vivo the activity of HBV-specific CD8 + T cells and were able to impair Th1 responses to HBcAg, by releasing increased amounts of IL-10. Several reports have highlighted the role of IL-10 as immunoregulatory cytokine in inflammatory responses [353], with preferential immunosuppressive properties, as well as potential stimulatory abilities under particular conditions. IL-10 gene promoter polymorphism has been shown to influence disease progression in patients with HBV chronic infection [354]. Recently, IL-10-IL10 receptor pathway has been shown to display a critical role in immune response, influencing the outcome of viral infection. The blockade of IL-10 receptor has been associated with the prevention of T cell exhaustion and the development of an immune response able to resolve a persistent viral infection.

References

[1]   Visvanathan K, Lewin SR. Immunopathogenesis: role of innate and adaptive immune responses. *Semin Liver Dis.* 2006; 26:104-115.

[2]   Lee WM. Hepatitis B virus infection. *N. Engl J Med* 1997; 337: 1733-1745.

[3]   Fattovich G, Giustina G, Schalm SW, Hadziyannis S, Sanchez-Tapias J, Almasio P, Christensen E, Krogsgaard K, Degos F, Carneiro de Moura M, et al. Occurrence of hepatocellular carcinoma and decompensation in western European patients with cirrhosis type B. The EUROHEP Study Group on Hepatitis B Virus and Cirrhosis. *Hepatology.* 1995; 21:77-82.

[4]   Di Marco V, Lo Iacono O, Camma C, Vaccaro A, Giunta M, Martorana G, Fuschi P, Almasio PL, Craxi A. The long-term course of chronic hepatitis B. *Hepatology.* 1999; 30:257-264.

[5]   Baumert TF, Thimme R, von Weizsacker F. Pathogenesis of hepatitis B virus infection. *World J Gastroenterol.* 2007; 13:82-90.

[6]   Chisari FV, Ferrari C, Mondelli MU. *Microb Pathog* 1989; 6: 311-325.

[7]   Mills CT, Lee E and Perrillo R. Relationship between histology, aminotransferase levels and viral replication in chronic hepatitis B. *Gastroenterology* 1990; 99: 519-524.

[8]   Chisari FV, Ferrari C. Hepatitis B virus immunophatogenesis. *Annu Rev Immunol* 1995; 13: 29-60.

[9]   Bertoletti A, Gehring AJ. The immune response during hepatitis B virus infection. *J Gen Virol.* 2006; 87: 1439-1449.

[10]   Whitton JL, Slifka MK, Liu F, Nussbaum AK, Whitmire JK. The regulation and maturation of antiviral immune responses. *Adv Virus Res.* 2004; 63:181-238.

[11]   Sharpe AH, Abbas AK. T-cell costimulation--biology, therapeutic potential, and challenges. *N Engl J Med.* 2006; 355:973-975.

[12]   Banchereau J, Steinman RM. Dendritic cells and the control of immunity. *Nature* 1998; 392: 245-251.

[13]   Lanzavecchia A and Sallustio F. Dynamics of T lymphocytes responses: intermediates, effectors and memory cells. *Science* 2000; 290: 92-97.

[14]   Doherty DG, O'Farrelly C. Innate and adaptive lymphoid cells in the human liver. *Immunol Rev.* 2000;174:5-20.

[15]   Moser M, Murphy KM. Dendritic cell regulation of TH1-TH2 development. *Nat Immunol.* 2000; 1:199-205.

[16]   Trinchieri G, Sher A. Cooperation of Toll-like receptor signals in innate immune defence. *Nat Rev Immunol.* 2007; 7:179-190.

[17]   Akira S. TLR signaling. *Curr Top Microbiol Immunol.* 2006; 311:1-16.

[18]   Barton GM. Viral recognition by Toll-like receptors. *Semin Immunol.* 2007; 19:33-40.

[19]   Macagno A, Napolitani G, Lanzavecchia A, Sallusto F. Duration, combination and timing: the signal integration model of dendritic cell activation. *Trends Immunol.* 2007; 28:227-233.

[20]   Granucci F, Foti M, Ricciardi-Castagnoli P. Dendritic cell biology. *Adv Immunol.* 2005; 88:193-233.

[21]   Dustin ML, Tseng SY, Varma R, Campi G. T cell-dendritic cell immunological synapses. *Curr Opin Immunol.* 2006;18:512-516.

[22]   Sanchez-Sanchez N, Riol-Blanco L, Rodriguez-Fernandez JL. The multiple personalities of the chemokine receptor CCR7 in dendritic cells. *J Immunol.* 2006;176:5153-5159.

[23]   Randolph GJ, Sanchez-Schmitz G, Angeli V. Factors and signals that govern the migration of dendritic cells via lymphatics: recent advances. *Springer Semin Immunopathol.* 2005;26:273-287.

[24]   Steinman RM, Hemmi H. Dendritic cells: translating innate to adaptive immunity. *Curr Top Microbiol Immunol.* 2006; 311:17-58.

[25]   de Jong EC, Smits HH, Kapsenberg ML. Dendritic cell-mediated T cell polarization. *Springer Semin Immunopathol.* 2005;26:289-307.

[26]   Jarrossay D, Napolitani G, Colonna M, Sallusto F, Lanzavecchia A. Specialization and complementarity in microbial molecule recognition by human myeloid and plasmacytoid dendritic cells. *Eur J Immunol.* 2001;31:3388-3393.

[27]   Kaisho T, Akira S. Regulation of dendritic cell function through toll-like receptors. *Curr Mol Med.* 2003;3:759-771.

[28]   Kadowaki N, Ho S, Antonenko S, Malefyt RW, Kastelein RA, Bazan F, Liu YJ. Subsets of human dendritic cell precursors express different toll-like receptors and respond to different microbial antigens. *J Exp Med.* 2001;194:863-869.

[29]   Moretta L, Ferlazzo G, Bottino C, Vitale M, Pende D, Mingari MC, Moretta A. Effector and regulatory events during natural killer-dendritic cell interactions. *Immunol Rev.* 2006;214:219-228.

[30]   Rossi M, Young JW. Human dendritic cells: potent antigen-presenting cells at the crossroads of innate and adaptive immunity. *J Immunol.* 2005;175:1373-1381.

[31]   Trinchieri G. Interleukin-12 and the regulation of innate resistance and adaptive immunity. *Nat Rev Immunol.* 2003;3:133-146.

[32]   Trinchieri G, Pflanz S, Kastelein RA. The IL-12 family of heterodimeric cytokines: new players in the regulation of T cell responses. *Immunity.* 2003; 19: 641-644.

[33]   Smits HH, van Beelen AJ, Hessle C, Westland R, de Jong E, Soeteman E, Wold A, Wierenga EA, Kapsenberg ML. Commensal Gram-negative bacteria prime human dendritic cells for enhanced IL-23 and IL-27 expression and enhanced Th1 development. *Eur J Immunol.* 2004; 34:1371-80.

[34]   Fujii S, Liu K, Smith C, Bonito AJ, Steinman RM. The linkage of innate to adaptive immunity via maturing dendritic cells in vivo requires CD40 ligation in addition to antigen presentation and CD80/86 costimulation. *J Exp Med.* 2004;199:1607-1618.

[35]   Ingulli E, Mondino A, Khoruts A, Jenkins MK. In vivo detection of dendritic cell antigen presentation to CD4(+) T cells. *J Exp Med.* 1997;185:2133-2141.

[36]   Andoniou CE, Andrews DM, Degli-Esposti MA. Natural killer cells in viral infection: more than just killers. *Immunol Rev.* 2006;214:239-250.

[37]   Papamichail M, Perez SA, Gritzapis AD, Baxevanis CN. Natural killer lymphocytes: biology, development, and function. *Cancer Immunol Immunother.* 2004;53:176-186.

[38]   French AR, Yokoyama WM. Natural killer cells and viral infections. *Curr Opin Immunol.* 2003; 15:45-51.

[39]   Di Santo JP. Natural killer cell developmental pathways: a question of balance. *Annu Rev Immunol.* 2006;24:257-86.

[40] Cooper MA, Fehniger TA, Turner SC, Chen KS, Ghaheri BA, Ghayur T, Carson WE, Caligiuri MA. Human natural killer cells: a unique innate immunoregulatory role for the CD56(bright) subset. *Blood.* 2001;97:3146-3151.

[41] Robertson MJ, Ritz J. Biology and clinical relevance of human natural killer cells. *Blood.* 1990;76:2421-2438.

[42] Vitale M, Della Chiesa M, Carlomagno S, Romagnani C, Thiel A, Moretta L, Moretta A. The small subset of CD56brightCD16- natural killer cells is selectively responsible for both cell proliferation and interferon-gamma production upon interaction with dendritic cells. *Eur J Immunol.* 2004;34:1715-1722.

[43] Berahovich RD, Lai NL, Wei Z, Lanier LL, Schall TJ. Evidence for NK cell subsets based on chemokine receptor expression. *J Immunol.* 2006;177:7833-7840.

[44] Moretta L, Biassoni R, Bottino C, Mingari MC, Moretta A. Natural killer cells: a mystery no more. *Scand J Immunol.* 2002;55:229-232.

[45] Biron CA, Nguyen KB, Pien GC, Cousens LP, Salazar-Mather TP. Natural killer cells in antiviral defense: function and regulation by innate cytokines. *Annu Rev Immunol.* 1999;17:189-220.

[46] Guidotti LG, Chisari FV. Noncytolytic control of viral infections by the innate and adaptive immune response. *Annu Rev Immunol.* 2001;19:65-91.

[47] Zhang C, Zhang J, Tian Z. The regulatory effect of natural killer cells: do "NK-reg cells" exist? *Cell Mol Immunol.* 2006;3:241-254.

[48] Joyce S. CD1d and natural T cells: how their properties jump-start the immune system. *Cell Mol Life Sci.* 2001;58:442-469.

[49] Kirwan SE, Burshtyn DN. Regulation of natural killer cell activity. *Curr Opin Immunol.* 2007;19:46-54.

[50] Moretta L, Ferlazzo G, Mingari MC, Melioli G, Moretta A. Human natural killer cell function and their interactions with dendritic cells. *Vaccine.* 2003; 21 Suppl 2:S38-42.

[51] Zitvogel L, Terme M, Borg C, Trinchieri G. Dendritic cell-NK cell cross-talk: regulation and physiopathology. *Curr Top Microbiol Immunol.* 2006;298:157-74.

[52] Zingoni A, Sornasse T, Cocks BG, Tanaka Y, Santoni A, Lanier LL. NK cell regulation of T cell-mediated responses. *Mol Immunol.* 2005;42:451-454.

[53] Exley MA, Koziel MJ. To be or not to be NKT: natural killer T cells in the liver. *Hepatology.* 2004;40:1033-1040.

[54] Kinjo Y, Kronenberg M. Valpha14i NKT cells are innate lymphocytes that participate in the immune response to diverse microbes. *J Clin Immunol.* 2005;25:522-533.

[55] Mercer JC, Ragin MJ, August A. Natural killer T cells: rapid responders controlling immunity and disease. *Int J Biochem Cell Biol.* 2005; 37:1337-1343

[56] Van Kaer L. NKT cells: T lymphocytes with innate effector functions. *Curr Opin Immunol.* 2007;19:354-364.

[57] Cui J, Shin T, Kawano T, Sato H, Kondo E, Toura I, Kaneko Y, Koseki H, Kanno M, Taniguchi M. Requirement for Valpha14 NKT cells in IL-12-mediated rejection of tumors. *Science.* 1997;278:1623-1626.

[58] Lantz O, Bendelac A. An invariant T cell receptor alpha chain is used by a unique subset of major histocompatibility complex class I-specific CD4+ and CD4-8- T cells in mice and humans. *J Exp Med.* 1994;180:1097-1106.

[59] Tsuji M. Glycolipids and phospholipids as natural CD1d-binding NKT cell ligands. *Cell Mol Life Sci.* 2006;63:1889-1898.

[60] Exley M, Garcia J, Wilson SB, Spada F, Gerdes D, Tahir SM, Patton KT, Blumberg RS, Porcelli S, Chott A, Balk SP. CD1d structure and regulation on human thymocytes, peripheral blood T cells, B cells and monocytes. *Immunology.* 2000;100:37-47.

[61] Durante-Mangoni E, Wang R, Shaulov A, He Q, Nasser I, Afdhal N, Koziel MJ, Exley MA. Hepatic CD1d expression in hepatitis C virus infection and recognition by resident proinflammatory CD1d-reactive T cells. *J Immunol.* 2004;173:2159-2166.

[62] Kronenberg M. Toward an understanding of NKT cell biology: progress and paradoxes. *Annu Rev Immunol.* 2005;23:877-900.

[63] Mercer JC, Ragin MJ, August A. Natural killer T cells: rapid responders controlling immunity and disease. *Int J Biochem Cell Biol.* 2005;37:1337-1343.

[64] Carnaud C, Lee D, Donnars O, Park SH, Beavis A, Koezuka Y, Bendelac A. Cutting edge: Cross-talk between cells of the innate immune system: NKT cells rapidly activate NK cells. *J Immunol.* 1999;163:4647-4650.

[65] Montoya CJ, Jie HB, Al-Harthi L, Mulder C, Patino PJ, Rugeles MT, Krieg AM, Landay AL, Wilson SB. Activation of plasmacytoid dendritic cells with TLR9 agonists initiates invariant NKT cell-mediated cross-talk with myeloid dendritic cells. *J Immunol.* 2006; 177:1028-1039.

[66] Eberl G, MacDonald HR. Selective induction of NK cell proliferation and cytotoxicity by activated NKT cells. *Eur J Immunol.* 2000;30:985-992.

[67] La Cava A, Van Kaer L, Fu-Dong-Shi. CD4+CD25+ Tregs and NKT cells: regulators regulating regulators.*Trends Immunol.* 2006;27:322-327.

[68] Zhang C, Zhang J, Tian Z. The regulatory effect of natural killer cells: do "NK-reg cells" exist? *Cell Mol Immunol.* 2006;3:241-54.

[69] Doherty PC. Cytotoxic T cell effector and memory function in viral immunity. *Curr Top Microbiol Immunol.* 1996;206:1-14.

[70] Klenerman P, Hill A. T cells and viral persistence: lessons from diverse infections. *Nat Immunol.* 2005;6:873-879.

[71] Al-Shanti N, Aldahoudi Z. Human purified CD8+ T cells: Ex vivo expansion model to generate a maximum yield of functional cytotoxic cells. *Immunol Invest.* 2007;36:85-104.

[72] Watson AR, Lee WT. Differences in signaling molecule organization between naive and memory CD4+ T lymphocytes. *J Immunol.* 2004;173:33-341.

[73] Appay V, Papagno L, Spina CA, Hansasuta P, King A, Jones L, Ogg GS, Little S, McMichael AJ, Richman DD, Rowland-Jones SL. Dynamics of T cell responses in HIV infection. *J Immunol.* 2002;168:3660-3666.

[74] Appay V, Zaunders JJ, Papagno L, Sutton J, Jaramillo A, Waters A, Easterbrook P, Grey P, Smith D, McMichael AJ, Cooper DA, Rowland-Jones SL, Kelleher AD. Characterization of CD4(+) CTLs ex vivo.*J Immunol.* 2002;168:5954-5958.

[75] Harari A, Vallelian F, Meylan PR, Pantaleo G. Functional heterogeneity of memory CD4 T cell responses in different conditions of antigen exposure and persistence. *J Immunol.* 2005;174:1037-1045.

[76] Sprent J, Surh CD. T cell memory. *Annu Rev Immunol.* 2002;20:551-579.

[77] Seder RA, Ahmed R Similarities and differences in CD4[+] and CD8[+] effector and memory T cell generation. *Nature Immunology* (2003) 4, 835 - 842.

[78] Wherry EJ, Teichgraber V, Becker TC, Masopust D, Kaech SM, Antia R, von Andrian UH, Ahmed R. Lineage relationship and protective immunity of memory CD8 T cell subsets. *Nat Immunol.* 2003;4:225-234.

[79] Lanzavecchia A, Sallusto F. Understanding the generation and function of memory T cell subsets. *Curr Opin Immunol.* 2005;17:326-332.

[80] Sallusto F, Lanzavecchia A. Exploring pathways for memory T cell generation. *J Clin Invest.* 2001;108:805-806.

[81]   Tan JT, Dudl E, LeRoy E, Murray R, Sprent J, Weinberg KI, Surh CD.
        IL-7 is critical for homeostatic proliferation and survival of naive T cells.
        Proc Natl Acad Sci U S A. 2001;98:8732-8737.

[82]   Tanchot C, Lemonnier FA, Perarnau B, Freitas AA, Rocha B. Differential
        requirements for survival and proliferation of CD8 naive or memory T
        cells. *Science.* 1997;276:2057-2062.

[83]   Nesic D, Vukmanovic S. MHC class I is required for peripheral
        accumulation of CD8+ thymic emigrants. *J Immunol.* 1998;160:3705-
        3712.

[84]   Takeda S, Rodewald HR, Arakawa H, Bluethmann H, Shimizu T. MHC
        class II molecules are not required for survival of newly generated CD4+
        T cells, but affect their long-term life span.*Immunity.* 1996;5:217-228.

[85]   Brocker T. Survival of mature CD4 T lymphocytes is dependent on major
        histocompatibility complex class II-expressing dendritic cells. *J Exp Med.*
        1997;186:1223-1232.

[86]   Schluns KS, Kieper WC, Jameson SC, Lefrancois L. Interleukin-7
        mediates the homeostasis of naive and memory CD8 T cells in vivo. *Nat
        Immunol.* 2000;1:426-432.

[87]   Lodolce JP, Boone DL, Chai S, Swain RE, Dassopoulos T, Trettin S, Ma
        A. IL-15 receptor maintains lymphoid homeostasis by supporting
        lymphocyte homing and proliferation. *Immunity.* 1998;9:669-676.

[88]   Kennedy MK, Glaccum M, Brown SN, Butz EA, Viney JL, Embers M,
        Matsuki N, Charrier K, Sedger L, Willis CR, Brasel K, Morrissey PJ,
        Stocking K, Schuh JC, Joyce S, Peschon JJ. Reversible defects in natural
        killer and memory CD8 T cell lineages in interleukin 15-deficient mice. *J
        Exp Med.* 2000 191:771-780.

[89]   Surh CD, Boyman O, Purton JF, Sprent J. Homeostasis of memory T
        cells. *Immunol Rev.* 2006; 211:154-163.

[90]   Sallusto F, Geginat J, Lanzavecchia A. Central memory and effector
        memory T cell subsets: function, generation, and maintenance. *Annu Rev
        Immunol.* 2004;22:745-763.

[91]   Harari A, Dutoit V, Cellerai C, Bart PA, Du Pasquier RA, Pantaleo G.
        Functional signatures of protective antiviral T-cell immunity in human
        virus infections. *Immunol Rev.* 2006;211:236-254.

[92]   Boyman O, Purton JF, Surh CD, Sprent J. Cytokines and T-cell
        homeostasis. *Curr Opin Immunol.* 2007;19:320-326.

[93] Kaech SM, Wherry EJ, Ahmed R. Effector and memory T-cell differentiation: implications for vaccine development. *Nat Rev Immunol.* 2002;2:251-262.

[94] Ahmed R, Gray D. Immunological memory and protective immunity: understanding their relation. *Science.* 1996;272:54-60.

[95] Appay V, Dunbar PR, Callan M, Klenerman P, Gillespie GM, Papagno L, Ogg GS, King A, Lechner F, Spina CA, Little S, Havlir DV, Richman DD, Gruener N, Pape G, Waters A, Easterbrook P, Salio M, Cerundolo V, McMichael AJ, Rowland-Jones SL. Memory CD8+ T cells vary in differentiation phenotype in different persistent virus infections. *Nat Med.* 2002;8:379-385.

[96] Ellefsen K, Harari A, Champagne P, Bart PA, Sekaly RP, Pantaleo G. Distribution and functional analysis of memory antiviral CD8 T cell responses in HIV-1 and cytomegalovirus infections. *Eur J Immunol.* 2002; 32:3756-3764.

[97] Pantaleo G, Harari A. Functional signatures in antiviral T-cell immunity for monitoring virus-associated diseases. *Nat Rev Immunol.* 2006;6:417-423.

[98] Paiardini M, Cervasi B, Albrecht H, Muthukumar A, Dunham R, Gordon S, Radziewicz H, Piedimonte G, Magnani M, Montroni M, Kaech SM, Weintrob A, Altman JD, Sodora DL, Feinberg MB, Silvestri G. Loss of CD127 expression defines an expansion of effector CD8+ T cells in HIV-infected individuals. *J Immunol.* 2005;174:2900-2909.

[99] Boutboul F, Puthier D, Appay V, Pelle O, Ait-Mohand H, Combadiere B, Carcelain G, Katlama C, Rowland-Jones SL, Debre P, Nguyen C, Autran B. Modulation of interleukin-7 receptor expression characterizes differentiation of CD8 T cells specific for HIV, EBV and CMV. *AIDS.* 2005;19:1981-1986.

[100] Campbell JJ, Murphy KE, Kunkel EJ, Brightling CE, Soler D, Shen Z, Boisvert J, Greenberg HB, Vierra MA, Goodman SB, Genovese MC, Wardlaw AJ, Butcher EC, Wu L. CCR7 expression and memory T cell diversity in humans. *J Immunol.* 2001;166:877-884.

[101] Wills MR, Carmichael AJ, Weekes MP, Mynard K, Okecha G, Hicks R, Sissons JG. Human virus-specific CD8+ CTL clones revert from CD45ROhigh to CD45RAhigh in vivo: CD45RAhighCD8+ T cells comprise both naive and memory cells. *J Immunol.* 1999;162:7080-7087.

[102] Hendriks J, Gravestein LA, Tesselaar K, van Lier RA, Schumacher TN, Borst J. CD27 is required for generation and long-term maintenance of T cell immunity. *Nat Immunol.* 2000;1:433-440.

[103] Sallusto F, Lenig D, Forster R, Lipp M, Lanzavecchia A. Two subsets of memory T lymphocytes with distinct homing potentials and effector functions. *Nature.* 1999;401:708-712.

[104] van Lier RA, ten Berge IJ, Gamadia LE. Human CD8(+) T-cell differentiation in response to viruses. *Nat Rev Immunol.* 2003;3:931-939.

[105] Palmer BE, Boritz E, Wilson CC. Effects of sustained HIV-1 plasma viremia on HIV-1 Gag-specific CD4+ T cell maturation and function. *J Immunol.* 2004;172:3337-3347

[106] Younes SA, Yassine-Diab B, Dumont AR, Boulassel MR, Grossman Z, Routy JP, Sekaly RP. HIV-1 viremia prevents the establishment of interleukin 2-producing HIV-specific memory CD4+ T cells endowed with proliferative capacity. *J Exp Med.* 2003;198:1909-1922.

[107] Mosmann TR, Cherwinski H, Bond MW, Giedlin MA, Coffman RL. Two types of murine helper T cell clone. I. Definition according to profiles of lymphokine activities and secreted proteins. *J Immunol.* 1986;136: 2348-2357.

[108] Kelso A. Th1 and Th2 subsets: paradigms lost? *Immunol Today.* 1995; 16: 374-379.

[109] Fiorentino DF, Bond MW, Mosmann TR. Two types of mouse T helper cell. IV. Th2 clones secrete a factor that inhibits cytokine production by Th1 clones. *J Exp Med.* 1989;170: 2081-2095.

[110] Fitch FW, McKisic MD, Lancki DW, Gajewski TF. Differential regulation of murine T lymphocyte subsets.*Annu Rev Immunol.* 1993; 11:29-48.

[111] Appay V. The physiological role of cytotoxic CD4(+) T-cells: the holy grail? *Clin Exp Immunol.* 2004;138:10-13.

[112] Appay V, Rowland-Jones SL. Lessons from the study of T-cell differentiation in persistent human virus infection. *Semin Immunol.* 2004; 16:205-212.

[113] Harari A, Petitpierre S, Vallelian F, Pantaleo G. Skewed representation of functionally distinct populations of virus-specific CD4 T cells in HIV-1-infected subjects with progressive disease: changes after antiretroviral therapy. *Blood.* 2004;103:966-972.

[114] Yue FY, Kovacs CM, Dimayuga RC, Parks P, Ostrowski MA. HIV-1-specific memory CD4+ T cells are phenotypically less mature than cytomegalovirus-specific memory CD4+ T cells. *J Immunol.* 2004; 172:2476-2486.

[115] Gamadia LE, Rentenaar RJ, van Lier RA, ten Berge IJ. Properties of CD4(+) T cells in human cytomegalovirus infection. *Hum Immunol.* 2004;65:486-492.

[116] Amyes E, Hatton C, Montamat-Sicotte D, Gudgeon N, Rickinson AB, McMichael AJ, Callan MF. Characterization of the CD4+ T cell response to Epstein-Barr virus during primary and persistent infection. *J Exp Med.* 2003;198:903-911.

[117] Aslan N, Yurdaydin C, Wiegand J, Greten T, Ciner A, Meyer MF, Heiken H, Kuhlmann B, Kaiser T, Bozkaya H, Tillmann HL, Bozdayi AM, Manns MP, Wedemeyer H. Cytotoxic CD4 T cells in viral hepatitis. *J Viral Hepat.* 2006;13:505-514.

[118] Vahlenkamp TW, Tompkins MB, Tompkins WA. The role of CD4+CD25+ regulatory T cells in viral infections. *Vet Immunol Immunopathol.* 2005;108:219-225.

[119] Suvas S, Kumaraguru U, Pack CD, Lee S, Rouse BT. CD4+CD25+ T cells regulate virus-specific primary and memory CD8+ T cell responses. *J Exp Med.* 2003;198:889-901.

[120] Mills KH, McGuirk P. Antigen-specific regulatory T cells--their induction and role in infection. *Semin Immunol.* 2004;16:107-117.

[121] Wherry EJ, Ahmed R. Memory CD8 T-cell differentiation during viral infection. *J Virol.* 2004;78:5535-5545.

[122] Wills MR, Carmichael AJ, Mynard K, Jin X, Weekes MP, Plachter B, Sissons JG. The human cytotoxic T-lymphocyte (CTL) response to cytomegalovirus is dominated by structural protein pp65: frequency, specificity, and T-cell receptor usage of pp65-specific CTL. *J Virol.* 1996;70:7569-7579.

[123] Callan MF, Tan L, Annels N, Ogg GS, Wilson JD, O'Callaghan CA, Steven N, McMichael AJ, Rickinson AB. Direct visualization of antigen-specific CD8+ T cells during the primary immune response to Epstein-Barr virus In vivo. *J Exp Med.* 1998;187:1395-1402.

[124] Riddell SR, Watanabe KS, Goodrich JM, Li CR, Agha ME, Greenberg PD. Restoration of viral immunity in immunodeficient humans by the adoptive transfer of T cell clones. *Science.* 1992;257:238-241.

[125] Guidotti LG, Ishikawa T, Hobbs MV, Matzke B, Schreiber R, Chisari FV. Intracellular inactivation of the hepatitis B virus by cytotoxic T lymphocytes. *Immunity.* 1996;4:25-36.

[126] Lechner F, Gruener NH, Urbani S, Uggeri J, Santantonio T, Kammer AR, Cerny A, Phillips R, Ferrari C, Pape GR, Klenerman P. CD8+ T lymphocyte responses are induced during acute hepatitis C virus infection but are not sustained. *Eur J Immunol.* 2000;30:2479-2487.

[127] Doherty PC. Cytotoxic T cell effector and memory function in viral immunity. *Curr Top Microbiol Immunol.* 1996;206:1-14.

[128] Klenerman P, Hill A. T cells and viral persistence: lessons from diverse infections. *Nat Immunol.* 2005;6:873-879.

[129] Harari A, Dutoit V, Cellerai C, Bart PA, Du Pasquier RA, Pantaleo G. Functional signatures of protective antiviral T-cell immunity in human virus infections. *Immunol Rev.* 2006;211:236-254.

[130] Sun JC, Williams MA, Bevan MJ. CD4+ T cells are required for the maintenance, not programming, of memory CD8+ T cells after acute infection. *Nat Immunol.* 2004;5:927-933.

[131] Mercado R, Vijh S, Allen SE, Kerksiek K, Pilip IM, Pamer EG. Early programming of T cell populations responding to bacterial infection. *J Immunol.* 2000;165:6833-6839.

[132] Wang B, Norbury CC, Greenwood R, Bennink JR, Yewdell JW, Frelinger JA. Multiple paths for activation of naive CD8+ T cells: CD4-independent help. *J Immunol.* 2001;167:1283-1289.

[133] Sun JC, Bevan MJ. Defective CD8 T cell memory following acute infection without CD4 T cell help. *Science.* 2003;300:339-342.

[134] Shedlock DJ, Shen H. Requirement for CD4 T cell help in generating functional CD8 T cell memory. *Science.* 2003;300:337-339.

[135] Sun JC, Bevan MJ. Cutting edge: long-lived CD8 memory and protective immunity in the absence of CD40 expression on CD8 T cells. *J Immunol.* 2004;172:3385-3389.

[136] Janssen EM, Lemmens EE, Wolfe T, Christen U, von Herrath MG, Schoenberger SP. CD4+ T cells are required for secondary expansion and memory in CD8+ T lymphocytes. *Nature.* 2003;421:852-856.

[137] Bourgeois C, Veiga-Fernandes H, Joret AM, Rocha B, Tanchot C. CD8 lethargy in the absence of CD4 help. *Eur J Immunol.* 2002;32:2199-2207.

[138] Mintern JD, Davey GM, Belz GT, Carbone FR, Heath WR. Cutting edge: precursor frequency affects the helper dependence of cytotoxic T cells. *J Immunol.* 2002;168:977-980.

[139] Dooms H, Kahn E, Knoechel B, Abbas AK. IL-2 induces a competitive survival advantage in T lymphocytes. *J Immunol.* 2004;172:5973-5979.

[140] Wherry EJ, Barber DL, Kaech SM, Blattman JN, Ahmed R. Antigen-independent memory CD8 T cells do not develop during chronic viral infection. *Proc Natl Acad Sci U S A.* 2004;101:16004-16009.

[141] Vezys V, Masopust D, Kemball CC, Barber DL, O'Mara LA, Larsen CP, Pearson TC, Ahmed R, Lukacher AE. Continuous recruitment of naive T cells contributes to heterogeneity of antiviral CD8 T cells during persistent infection. J *Exp Med.* 2006;203:2263-2269.

[142] Barber DL, Wherry EJ, Masopust D, Zhu B, Allison JP, Sharpe AH, Freeman GJ, Ahmed R. Restoring function in exhausted CD8 T cells during chronic viral infection. *Nature.* 2006;439:682-687.

[143] Kaech SM, Tan JT, Wherry EJ, Konieczny BT, Surh CD, Ahmed R. Selective expression of the interleukin 7 receptor identifies effector CD8 T cells that give rise to long-lived memory cells. *Nat Immunol.* 2003;4:1191-1198.

[144] Boutboul F, Puthier D, Appay V, Pelle O, Ait-Mohand H, Combadiere B, Carcelain G, Katlama C, Rowland-Jones SL, Debre P, Nguyen C, Autran B. Modulation of interleukin-7 receptor expression characterizes differentiation of CD8 T cells specific for HIV, EBV and CMV. *AIDS.* 2005;19:1981-1986.

[145] Colle JH, Moreau JL, Fontanet A, Lambotte O, Joussemet M, Delfraissy JF, Theze J. CD127 expression and regulation are altered in the memory CD8 T cells of HIV-infected patients--reversal by highly active anti-retroviral therapy (HAART). *Clin Exp Immunol.* 2006;143:398-403.

[146] Paiardini M, Cervasi B, Albrecht H, Muthukumar A, Dunham R, Gordon S, Radziewicz H, Piedimonte G, Magnani M, Montroni M, Kaech SM, Weintrob A, Altman JD, Sodora DL, Feinberg MB, Silvestri G. Loss of CD127 expression defines an expansion of effector CD8+ T cells in HIV-infected individuals. *J Immunol.* 2005;174:2900-2909.

[147] Fuller MJ, Hildeman DA, Sabbaj S, Gaddis DE, Tebo AE, Shang L, Goepfert PA, Zajac AJ. Cutting edge: emergence of CD127high functionally competent memory T cells is compromised by high viral loads and inadequate T cell help. *J Immunol.* 2005;174:5926-5930.

[148] van Leeuwen EM, de Bree GJ, Remmerswaal EB, Yong SL, Tesselaar K, ten Berge IJ, van Lier RA. IL-7 receptor alpha chain expression distinguishes functional subsets of virus-specific human CD8+ T cells. *Blood.* 2005;106:2091-2098.

[149] Sabbaj S, Heath SL, Bansal A, Vohra S, Kilby JM, Zajac AJ, Goepfert PA. Functionally competent antigen-specific CD127(hi) memory CD8+ T cells are preserved only in HIV-infected individuals receiving early treatment. *J Infect Dis.* 2007;195:108-117.

[150] Lanzavecchia A, Bernasconi N, Traggiai E, Ruprecht CR, Corti D, Sallusto F. Understanding and making use of human memory B cells. *Immunol Rev.* 2006;211:303-309.

[151] Cassell DJ, Schwartz RH. A quantitative analysis of antigen-presenting cell function: activated B cells stimulate naive CD4 T cells but are inferior to dendritic cells in providing costimulation. *J Exp Med.* 1994;180:1829-1840.

[152] Rivera A, Chen CC, Ron N, Dougherty JP, Ron Y. Role of B cells as antigen-presenting cells in vivo revisited: antigen-specific B cells are essential for T cell expansion in lymph nodes and for systemic T cell responses to low antigen concentrations. *Int Immunol.* 2001;13:1583-1593.

[153] Harris DP, Goodrich S, Mohrs K, Mohrs M, Lund FE. Cutting edge: the development of IL-4-producing B cells (B effector 2 cells) is controlled by IL-4, IL-4 receptor alpha, and Th2 cells. *J Immunol.* 2005;175:7103-7107.

[154] Harris DP, Haynes L, Sayles PC, Duso DK, Eaton SM, Lepak NM, Johnson LL, Swain SL, Lund FE. Reciprocal regulation of polarized cytokine production by effector B and T cells. *Nat Immunol.* 2000;1:475-482.

[155] Mills DM, Cambier JC. B lymphocyte activation during cognate interactions with CD4+ T lymphocytes: molecular dynamics and immunologic consequences. *Semin Immunol.* 2003;15:325-329.

[156] Garside P, Ingulli E, Merica RR, Johnson JG, Noelle RJ, Jenkins MK. Visualization of specific B and T lymphocyte interactions in the lymph node. *Science.* 1998;281:96-99.

[157] McHeyzer-Williams LJ, Malherbe LP, McHeyzer-Williams MG. Checkpoints in memory B-cell evolution. *Immunol Rev.* 2006;211:255-268.

[158] MacLennan IC, Gulbranson-Judge A, Toellner KM, Casamayor-Palleja M, Chan E, Sze DM, Luther SA, Orbea HA. The changing preference of T and B cells for partners as T-dependent antibody responses develop. *Immunol Rev.* 1997;156:53-66.

[159]   Bishop GA, Hostager BS. B lymphocyte activation by contact-mediated interactions with T lymphocytes. *Curr Opin Immunol.* 2001;13:278-285.

[160]   Linton PJ, Harbertson J, Bradley LM. A critical role for B cells in the development of memory CD4 cells. *J Immunol.* 2000;165:5558-5565.

[161]   Bradley LM, Harbertson J, Freschi GC, Kondrack R, Linton PJ. Regulation of development and function of memory CD4 subsets. *Immunol Res.* 2000;2:149-158.

[162]   Galli G, Pittoni P, Tonti E, Malzone C, Uematsu Y, Tortoli M, Maione D, Volpini G, Finco O, Nuti S, Tavarini S, Dellabona P, Rappuoli R, Casorati G, Abrignani S. Invariant NKT cells sustain specific B cell responses and memory. *Proc Natl Acad Sci U S A.* 2007;104:3984-3989.

[163]   McHeyzer-Williams LJ, Malherbe LP, McHeyzer-Williams MG. Helper T cell-regulated B cell immunity. *Curr Top Microbiol Immunol.* 2006;311:59-83.

[164]   Parker DC. T cell-dependent B cell activation. *Annu Rev Immunol.* 1993;11:331-360.

[165]   Ruprecht CR, Lanzavecchia A. Toll-like receptor stimulation as a third signal required for activation of human naive B cells. *Eur J Immunol.* 2006;36:810-816.

[166]   MacPherson G, Kushnir N, Wykes M. Dendritic cells, B cells and the regulation of antibody synthesis. *Immunol Rev.* 1999;172:325-334.

[167]   Colino J, Shen Y, Snapper CM. Dendritic cells pulsed with intact Streptococcus pneumoniae elicit both protein- and polysaccharide-specific immunoglobulin isotype responses in vivo through distinct mechanisms. *J Exp Med.* 2002;195:1-13.

[168]   Rajewsky K. Clonal selection and learning in the antibody system. *Nature.* 1996;381:751-758.

[169]   Nassal M. Hepatitis B virus replication: novel roles for virus-host interactions. *Intervirology.* 1999;42:100-116.

[170]   Beck J, Nassal M. Hepatitis B virus replication. World J Gastroenterol. 2007;13:48-64.

[171]   Summers J, Mason WS. Replication of the genome of a hepatitis B--like virus by reverse transcription of an RNA intermediate. *Cell.* 1982;29:403-415.

[172]   Tong SP, Diot C, Gripon P, Li J, Vitvitski L, Trepo C, Guguen-Guillouzo C. In vitro replication competence of a cloned hepatitis B virus variant with a nonsense mutation in the distal pre-C region. *Virology.* 1991;181:733-737.

[173] Lenschow DJ, Walunas TL, Bluestone JA. CD28/B7 system of T cell costimulation. *Annu Rev Immunol* 1996; 14: 233-258.

[174] Bertoletti A, Ferrari C, Fiaccadori F, Penna A, Margolskee R, Schlicht HJ, Fowler P, Guilhot S, Chisari FV. HLA class I-restricted human cytotoxic T cells recognize endogenously synthesized hepatitis B virus nucleocapsid antigen. *Proc Natl Acad Sci U S A.* 1991; 88:10445-10449.

[175] Milich DR, McLachlan A, Thornton GB, Hughes JL. Antibody production to the nucleocapsid and envelope of the hepatitis B virus primed by a single synthetic T cell site. *Nature* 1987;329:547-549.

[176] Penna A, Del Prete G, Cavalli A, Bertoletti A, D'Elios MM, Sorrentino R, D'Amato M, Boni C, Pilli M, Fiaccadori F, Ferrari C. Predominant T-helper 1 cytokine profile of hepatitis B virus nucleocapsid-specific T cells in acute self-limited hepatitis B. *Hepatology.* 1997;25:1022-1027.

[177] Perrillo RP. Acute flares in chronic hepatitis B: the natural and unnatural history of an immunologically mediated liver disease. *Gastroenterology.* 2001;120:1009-1022.

[178] Seeff LB, Koff RS. Evolving concepts of the clinical and serologic consequences of hepatitis B virus infection. *Semin Liver Dis.* 1986;6:11-22.

[179] Tsai SL, Chen PJ, Lai MY, Yang PM, Sung JL, Huang JH, Hwang LH, Chang TH, Chen DS. Acute exacerbations of chronic type B hepatitis are accompanied by increased T cell responses to hepatitis B core and e antigens. Implications for hepatitis B e antigen seroconversion. *J Clin Invest.* 1992;89:87-96.

[180] Lau GK, Suri D, Liang R, Rigopoulou EI, Thomas MG, Mullerova I, Nanji A, Yuen ST, Williams R, Naoumov NV. Resolution of chronic hepatitis B and anti-HBs seroconversion in humans by adoptive transfer of immunity to hepatitis B core antigen. *Gastroenterology.* 2002;122:614-624.

[181] Lau GK, Liang R, Lee CK, Yuen ST, Hou J, Lim WL, Williams R. Clearance of persistent hepatitis B virus infection in Chinese bone marrow transplant recipients whose donors were anti-hepatitis B core- and anti-hepatitis B surface antibody-positive. *J Infect Dis.* 1998;178:1585-1591.

[182] Missale G, Redeker A, Person J, Fowler P, Guilhot S, Schlicht HJ, Ferrari C, Chisari FV. HLA-A31- and HLA-Aw68-restricted cytotoxic T cell responses to a single hepatitis B virus nucleocapsid epitope during acute viral hepatitis. *J Exp Med.* 1993;177:751-762.

[183] Bertoletti A, Chisari FV, Penna A, Guilhot S, Galati L, Missale G, Fowler
       P, Schlicht HJ, Vitiello A, Chesnut RC, et al. Definition of a minimal
       optimal cytotoxic T-cell epitope within the hepatitis B virus nucleocapsid
       protein. *J Virol.* 1993;67:2376-2380.
[184] Ferrari C, Bertoletti A, Penna A, Cavalli A, Valli A, Missale G, Pilli M,
       Fowler P, Giuberti T, Chisari FV, et al. Identification of immunodominant
       T cell epitopes of the hepatitis B virus nucleocapsid antigen. *J Clin Invest.*
       1991;88:214-222.
[185] Milich DR, Schodel F, Hughes JL, Jones JE, Peterson DL. The hepatitis B
       virus core and e antigens elicit different Th cell subsets: antigen structure
       can affect Th cell phenotype. *J Virol.* 1997; 71:2192-2201.
[186] Milich DR, McLachlan A. The nucleocapsid of hepatitis B virus is both a
       T-cell-independent and a T-cell-dependent antigen. *Science.* 1986 Dec
       12;234(4782):1398-401.
[187] Carson DA, Raz E. Oligonucleotide adjuvants for T helper 1 (Th1)-
       specific vaccination. *J Exp Med.* 1997;186:1621-1622.
[188] Chu RS, Targoni OS, Krieg AM, Lehmann PV, Harding CV. CpG
       oligodeoxynucleotides act as adjuvants that switch on T helper 1 (Th1)
       immunity. *J Exp Med.* 1997;186:1623-1631.
[189] Riedl P, Stober D, Oehninger C, Melber K, Reimann J, Schirmbeck R.
       Priming Th1 immunity to viral core particles is facilitated by trace
       amounts of RNA bound to its arginine-rich. domain. *J Immunol.*
       2002;168:4951-4959.
[190] Milich DR, Peterson DL, Schodel F, Jones JE, Hughes JL.. Preferential
       recognition of hepatitis B nucleocapsid antigens by Th1 or Th2 is epitope
       and major histocompatibility complex dependent. *J Virol* 1995; 69: 2776-
       2785.
[191] Milich DR, Schodel F, Peterson DL, Jones JE, Hughes JL.
       Characterization of self-reactive T cells that evade tolerance in hepatitis B
       e antigen transgenic mice. *Eur J Immunol.* 1995;25:1663-1672.
[192] Milich DR, Chen MK, Hughes JL, Jones JE. The secreted hepatitis B
       precore antigen can modulate the immune response to the nucleocapsid: a
       mechanism for persistence. *J Immunol.* 1998;160:2013-2021.
[193] Milich DR. Influence of T-helper cell subsets and crossregulation in
       hepatitis B virus infection. *J Viral Hepat.* 1997;4 Suppl 2:48-59.
[194] Ferrari C, Mondelli MU, Penna A, Fiaccadori F, Chisari FV. Functional
       characterization of cloned intrahepatic, hepatitis B virus nucleoprotein-
       specific helper T cell lines. *J Immunol.* 1987;139:539-44.

[195] Barnaba V, Franco A, Alberti A, Balsano C, Benvenuto R, Balsano F. Recognition of hepatitis B virus envelope proteins by liver-infiltrating T lymphocytes in chronic HBV infection. *J Immunol.* 1989;143:2650-2655.

[196] Barnaba V, Franco A, Paroli M, Benvenuto R, De Petrillo G, Burgio VL, Santilio I, Balsano C, Bonavita MS, Cappelli G, et al. Selective expansion of cytotoxic T lymphocytes with a CD4+CD56+ surface phenotype and a T helper type 1 profile of cytokine secretion in the liver of patients chronically infected with Hepatitis B virus. *J Immunol.* 1994;152:3074-3087.

[197] Bertoletti A, D'Elios MM, Boni C, De Carli M, Zignego AL, Durazzo M, Missale G, Penna A, Fiaccadori F, Del Prete G, Ferrari C. Different cytokine profiles of intraphepatic T cells in chronic hepatitis B and hepatitis C virus infections. *Gastroenterology.* 1997;112:193-199.

[198] Visvanathan K, Skinner NA, Thompson AJ, Riordan SM, Sozzi V, Edwards R, Rodgers S, Kurtovic J, Chang J, Lewin S, Desmond P, Locarnini S. Regulation of Toll-like receptor-2 expression in chronic hepatitis B by the precore protein. *Hepatology.* 2007;45:102-110.

[199] Maruyama T, McLachlan A, Iino S, Koike K, Kurokawa K, Milich DR. The serology of chronic hepatitis B infection revisited. *J Clin Invest.* 1993;91:2586-2595.

[200] Samuel D, Muller R, Alexander G, Fassati L, Ducot B, Benhamou JP, Bismuth H. Liver transplantation in European patients with the hepatitis B surface antigen. *N Engl J Med.* 1993;329:1842-1847.

[201] Wainwright RB, McMahon BJ, Bulkow LR, Hall DB, Fitzgerald MA, Harpster AP, Hadler SC, Lanier AP, Heyward WL. Duration of immunogenicity and efficacy of hepatitis B vaccine in a Yupik Eskimo population. *JAMA.* 1989;261:2362-2366.

[202] Bocher WO, Galun E, Marcus H, Daudi N, Terkieltaub D, Shouval D, Lohr HF, Reisner Y. Reduced hepatitis B virus surface antigen-specific Th1 helper cell frequency of chronic HBV carriers is associated with a failure to produce antigen-specific antibodies in the trimera mouse. *Hepatology.* 2000;31: 480-487.

[203] Rehermann B, Fowler P, Sidney J, Person J, Redeker A, Brown M, Moss B, Sette A, Chisari FV. The cytotoxic T lymphocyte response to multiple hepatitis B virus polymerase epitopes during and after acute viral hepatitis. *J Exp Med.* 1995;181:1047-1058

[204]   Mizukoshi E, Sidney J, Livingston B, Ghany M, Hoofnagle JH, Sette A, Rehermann B. Cellular immune responses to the hepatitis B virus polymerase. *J Immunol.* 2004;173:5863-5871.

[205]   Jung MC, Stemler M, Weimer T, Spengler U, Dohrmann J, Hoffmann R, Eichenlaub D, Eisenburg J, Paumgartner G, Riethmuller G, et al. Immune response of peripheral blood mononuclear cells to HBx-antigen of hepatitis B virus. *Hepatology.* 1991;13:637-643.

[206]   Bartenschlager R, Schaller H. The amino-terminal domain of the hepadnaviral P-gene encodes the terminal protein (genome-linked protein) believed to prime reverse transcription. *EMBO J.* 1988;7:4185-4192.

[207]   Andus T, Bauer J, Gerok W. Effects of cytokines on the liver. *Hepatology.* 1991;13:364-375.

[208]   Chisari FV. Cytotoxic T cells and viral hepatitis. *J Clin Invest.* 1997;99:1472-1477.

[209]   Hsu HY, Chang MH Ni YH et al. Cytochine release of peripheral blood mononuclear cells in children with chronic hepatitis B virus infection. *J Pediatr Gastroenter Nutr* 1999; 29: 540-545.

[210]   Mogensen TH, Paludan SR. Molecular pathways in virus-induced cytokine production. *Microbiol Mol Biol Rev.* 2001;65:131-150.

[211]   Jung MC, Pape GR. Immunology of hepatitis B infection. *Lancet Infect Dis.* 2002;2:43-50.

[212]   Vingerhoets J, Michielsen P, Vanham G, Bosmans E, Paulij W, Ramon A, Pelckmans P, Kestens L, Leroux-Roels G. HBV-specific lymphoproliferative and cytokine responses in patients with chronic hepatitis B. *J Hepatol.* 1998;28:8-16.

[213]   Gonzalez-Amaro R, Garcia-Monzon C, Garcia-Buey L, Moreno-Otero R, Alonso JL, Yague E, Pivel JP, Lopez-Cabrera M, Fernandez-Ruiz E, Sanchez-Madrid F. Induction of tumor necrosis factor alpha production by human hepatocytes in chronic viral hepatitis. *J Exp Med.* 1994;179:841-848.

[214]   Lee Y, Park US, Choi I, Yoon SK, Park YM, Lee YI. Human interleukin 6 gene is activated by hepatitis B virus-X protein in human hepatoma cells. *Clin Cancer Res.* 1998;4:1711-1717.

[215]   Chen HS, Kaneko S, Girones R, Anderson RW, Hornbuckle WE, Tennant BC, Cote PJ, Gerin JL., Purcell RH, Miller RH. The woodchuck hepatitis virus X gene is important for establishment of virus infection in woodchucks. *J Virol.* 1993;67:1218-1226.

[216] Zoulim F, Saputelli J, Seeger C. Woodchuck hepatitis virus X protein is required for viral infection in vivo. *J Virol.* 1994;68:2026-2030.

[217] Henkler F, Hoare J, Waseem N, Goldin RD, McGarvey MJ, Koshy R, King IA. Intracellular localization of the hepatitis B virus HBx protein. *J Gen Virol.* 2001;82:871-882.

[218] Raney AK, Johnson JL, Palmer CN, McLachlan A. Members of the nuclear receptor superfamily regulate transcription from the hepatitis B virus nucleocapsid promoter. *J Virol.* 1997;71:1058-1071.

[219] Lin Y, Tang H, Nomura T, Dorjsuren D, Hayashi N, Wei W, Ohta T, Roeder R, Murakami S. The hepatitis B virus X protein is a co-activator of activated transcription that modulates the transcription machinery and distal binding activators. *J Biol Chem.* 1998;273:27097-27103.

[220] Balsano C, Avantaggiati ML, Natoli G, De Marzio E, Will H, Perricaudet M, Levrero M. Full-length and truncated versions of the hepatitis B virus (HBV) X protein (pX) transactivate the cmyc protooncogene at the transcriptional level. *Biochem Biophys Res Commun.* 1991;176:985-992.

[221] Su F, Schneider RJ. Hepatitis B virus HBx protein sensitizes cells to apoptotic killing by tumor necrosis factor. alpha. *Proc Natl Acad Sci U S A.* 1997;94:8744-8749.

[222] Natoli G, Avantaggiati ML, Chirillo P, Puri PL, Ianni A, Balsano C, Levrero M. Ras- and Raf-dependent activation of c-jun transcriptional activity by the hepatitis B virus transactivator pX. *Oncogene.* 1994;9:2837-2843.

[223] Cross JC, Wen P, Rutter WJ. Transactivation by hepatitis B virus X protein is promiscuous and dependent on mitogen-activated cellular serine/threonine kinases. *Proc Natl Acad Sci U S A.* 1993;90:8078-8082.

[224] Benn J, Schneider RJ. Hepatitis B virus HBx protein activates Ras-GTP complex formation and establishes a Ras, Raf, MAP kinase signaling cascade. *Proc Natl Acad Sci U S A.* 1994;91:10350-10354.

[225] Klein NP, Schneider RJ. Activation of Src family kinases by hepatitis B virus HBx protein and coupled signaling to Ras. *Mol Cell Biol.* 1997; 17:6427-6436.

[226] Baeuerle PA. The inducible transcription activator NF-kappa B: regulation by distinct protein subunits. *Biochim Biophys Acta.* 1991;1072:63-80.

[227] Ohno H, Kaneko S, Kobayashi K, Murakami S. Human hepatitis B virus enhancer 1 is responsive to human interleukin-6. *J Med Virol.* 1997;52:413-418.

[228] Shaul Y, Rutter WJ, Laub O. A human hepatitis B viral enhancer element. *EMBO J.* 1985; 4:427-430.

[229] Dikstein R, Faktor O, Ben-Levy R, Shaul Y. Functional organization of the hepatitis B virus enhancer. *Mol Cell Biol.* 1990;10:3683-3689.

[230] Chen M, Hieng S, Qian X, Costa R, Ou JH. Regulation of hepatitis B virus ENI enhancer activity by hepatocyte-enriched transcription factor HNF3. *Virology.* 1994;205:127-132.

[231] Ohno H, Kaneko S, Lin Y, Kobayashi K, Murakami S. Human hepatitis B virus X protein augments the DNA binding of nuclear factor for IL-6 through its basic-leucine zipper domain. *J Med Virol.* 1999;58:11-18.

[232] Gutman A, Wasylyk C, Wasylyk B. Cell-specific regulation of oncogene-responsive sequences of the c-fos promoter. *Mol Cell Biol.* 1991;11:5381-5387.

[233] Murakami S, Cheong J, Ohno S, Matsushima K, Kaneko S. Transactivation of human hepatitis B virus X protein, HBx, operates through a mechanism distinct from protein kinase C and okadaic acid activation pathways. *Virology.* 1994;199:243-246.

[234] Akira S, Isshiki H, Sugita T, Tanabe O, Kinoshita S, Nishio Y, Nakajima T, Hirano T, Kishimoto T. A nuclear factor for IL-6 expression (NF-IL6) is a member of a C/EBP family. *EMBO J.* 1990;9:1897-1906.

[235] Waris G, Siddiqui A. Interaction between STAT-3 and HNF-3 leads to the activation of liver-specific hepatitis B virus enhancer 1 function. *J Virol.* 2002;76:2721-2729.

[236] Kakumu S, Fukatsu A, Shinagawa T, Kurokawa S, Kusakabe A. Localisation of intrahepatic interleukin 6 in patients with acute and chronic liver disease. *J Clin Pathol.* 1992;45:408-411.

[237] Kakumu S, Shinagawa T, Ishikawa T, Yoshioka K, Wakita T, Ito Y, Takayanagi M, Ida N. Serum interleukin 6 levels in patients with chronic hepatitis B. *Am J Gastroenterol.* 1991;86:1804-1808.

[238] Mahe Y, Mukaida N, Kuno K, Akiyama M, Ikeda N, Matsushima K, Murakami S. Hepatitis B virus X protein transactivates human interleukin-8 gene through acting on nuclear factor kB and CCAAT/enhancer-binding protein-like cis-elements. *J Biol Chem.* 1991;266:13759-13763.

[239] Wieland SF, Chisari FV. Stealth and cunning: hepatitis B and hepatitis C viruses. *J Virol.* 2005;79: 9369-9380.

[240] Guidotti LG, Matzke B, Schaller H, Chisari FV. High-level hepatitis B virus replication in transgenic mice. *J Virol.* 1995;69:6158-6169.

[241] Altman JD, Moss PAH, Goulder PJR et al Phenotypic analysis of antigen-specific T lymphocytes. *Science* 1996; 274:94-96.

[242] Ogg GS, McMichael AJ. HLA-peptide tetrameric complexes. *Curr Opin Immunol* 1998; 10: 393-396.

[243] Maini MK, Boni C, Ogg GS, King AS, Reignat S, Lee CK, Larrubia JR, Webster GJ, McMichael AJ, Ferrari C, Williams R, Vergani D, Bertoletti A. Direct ex vivo analysis of hepatitis B virus-specific CD8(+) T cells associated with the control of infection. *Gastroenterology.* 1999;117:1386-1396.

[244] Penna A, Chisari F, Bertoletti A Cytotoxic T lymphocytes recognize an HLA-A2 restricted epitope within the hepatitis B virus nucleocapsid antigen. *J Exp Med* 1991; 174:1565-1570.

[245] Alexander-Miller MA, Leggatt GR, Sarin A, Berzofsky JA. Role of antigen, CD8, and cytotoxic T lymphocyte (CTL) avidity in high dose antigen induction of apoptosis of effector CTL. *J Exp Med.* 1996;184:485-492.

[246] Mondelli M, Vergani GM, Alberti A, Vergani D, Portmann B, Eddleston AL, Williams R. Specificity of T lymphocyte cytotoxicity to autologous hepatocytes in chronic hepatitis B virus infection: evidence that T cells are directed against HBV core antigen expressed on hepatocytes. *J Immunol.* 1982;129:2773-2778.

[247] Farza H, Hadchouel M, Scotto J, Tiollais P, Babinet C, Pourcel C. Replication and gene expression of hepatitis B virus in a transgenic mouse that contains the complete viral genome. *J Virol.* 1988;62:4144-4152.

[248] Araki K, Miyazaki J, Hino O, Tomita N, Chisaka O, Matsubara K, Yamamura K. Expression and replication of hepatitis B virus genome in transgenic mice. *Proc Natl Acad Sci U S A.* 1989;86:207-211.

[249] Moriyama T, Guilhot S, Klopchin K, Moss B, Pinkert CA, Palmiter RD, Brinster RL, Kanagawa O, Chisari FV. Immunobiology and pathogenesis of hepatocellular injury in hepatitis B virus transgenic mice. *Science.* 1990;248:361-364.

[250] Ando K, Moriyama T, Guidotti LG, Wirth S, Schreiber RD, Schlicht HJ, Huang SN, Chisari FV. Mechanisms of class I restricted immunopathology. A transgenic mouse model of fulminant hepatitis. *J Exp Med.* 1993;178:1541-1554.

[251] Ando K, Guidotti LG, Wirth S, Ishikawa T, Missale G, Moriyama T, Schreiber RD, Schlicht HJ, Huang SN, Chisari FV. Class I-restricted cytotoxic T lymphocytes are directly cytopathic for their target cells in vivo. *J Immunol.* 1994;152:3245-3253.

[252] Guidotti LG, Ando K, Hobbs MV, Ishikawa T, Runkel L, Schreiber RD, Chisari FV. Cytotoxic T lymphocytes inhibit hepatitis B virus gene expression by a noncytolytic mechanism in transgenic mice. *Proc Natl Acad Sci U S A.* 1994;91:3764-3768.

[253] Gilles PN, Fey G, Chisari FV. Tumor necrosis factor alpha negatively regulates hepatitis B virus gene expression in transgenic mice. *J Virol.* 1992;66:3955-3960.

[254] Guidotti LG, Guilhot S, Chisari FV. Interleukin-2 and alpha/beta interferon down-regulate hepatitis B virus gene expression in vivo by tumor necrosis factor-dependent and -independent pathways. *J Virol.* 1994;68:1265-1270.

[255] Guidotti LG, Chisari FV. Noncytolytic control of viral infections by the innate and adaptive immune response. *Annu Rev Immunol.* 2001;19:65-91.

[256] Guilhot S, Guidotti LG, Chisari FV. Interleukin-2 downregulates hepatitis B virus gene expression in transgenic mice by a posttranscriptional mechanism. *J Virol.* 1993;67:7444-7449.

[257] Kajino K, Jilbert AR, Saputelli J, Aldrich CE, Cullen J, Mason WS. Woodchuck hepatitis virus infections: very rapid recovery after a prolonged viremia and infection of virtually every hepatocyte. *J Virol.* 1994;68:5792-5803.

[258] Jilbert AR, Wu TT, England JM, Hall PM, Carp NZ, O'Connell AP, Mason WS. Rapid resolution of duck hepatitis B virus infections occurs after massive hepatocellular involvement. *J Virol.* 1992;66:1377-1388.

[259] Jilbert AR, Botten JA, Miller DS, Bertram EM, Hall PM, Kotlarski J, Burrell CJ. Characterization of age- and dose-related outcomes of duck hepatitis B virus infection. *Virology.* 1998;244:273-282.Bertoletti A, Costanzo A, Chisari FV, Levrero M, Artini M, Sette A, Penna A, Giuberti T, Fiaccadori F, Ferrari C. Cytotoxic T lymphocyte response to a wild type hepatitis B virus epitope in patients chronically infected by variant viruses carrying substitutions within the epitope. *J Exp Med.* 1994;180:933-943.

[261] Ferrari C, Penna A, Giuberti T, Tong MJ, Ribera E, Fiaccadori F, Chisari FV. Intrahepatic, nucleocapsid antigen-specific T cells in chronic active hepatitis B. *J Immunol.* 1987;139:2050-2058.

[262] Ferrari C, Penna A, Sansoni P, Giuberti T, Neri TM, Chisari FV, Fiaccadori F. Selective sensitization of peripheral blood T lymphocytes to hepatitis B core antigen in patients with chronic active hepatitis type B. Clin Exp Immunol. 1986;66:497-506.

[263] Rehermann B. Immunopathogenesis of viral hepatitis. *Baillieres Clin Gastroenterol.* 1996;10:483-500.

[264] Penna A, Artini M, Cavalli A, Levrero M, Bertoletti A, Pilli M, Chisari FV, Rehermann B, Del Prete G, Fiaccadori F, Ferrari C. Long-lasting memory T cell responses following self-limited acute hepatitis B. *J Clin Invest.* 1996;98:1185-1194.

[265] Jung MC, Hartmann B, Gerlach JT et al. Virus-specific lymphokine production differs quantitatively but not qualitatively in acute and chronic hepatitis B infection. *Virology* 1999; 261: 165-172.

[266] Nakamura I, Nupp JT, Cowlen M, Hall WC, Tennant BC, Casey JL, Gerin JL, Cote PJ. Pathogenesis of experimental neonatal woodchuck hepatitis virus infection: chronicity as an outcome of infection is associated with a diminished acute hepatitis that is temporally deficient for the expression of interferon gamma and tumor necrosis factor-alpha messenger RNAs. *Hepatology.* 2001;33:439-447.

[267] Guo JT, Zhou H, Liu C, Aldrich C, Saputelli J, Whitaker T, Barrasa MI, Mason WS, Seeger C. Apoptosis and regeneration of hepatocytes during recovery from transient hepadnavirus infections. *J Virol.* 2000;74:1495-1505.

[268] Guidotti LG, Rochford R, Chung J, Shapiro M, Purcell R, Chisari FV. Viral clearance without destruction of infected cells during acute HBV infection. *Science.* 1999;284:825-829.

[269] Wieland SF, Spangenberg HC, Thimme R, Purcell RH, Chisari FV. Expansion and contraction of the hepatitis B virus transcriptional template in infected chimpanzees. *Proc Natl Acad Sci U S A.* 2004;101:2129-2134.

[270] Takehara T, Suzuki T, Ohkawa K, Hosui A, Jinushi M, Miyagi T, Tatsumi T, Kanazawa Y, Hayashi N. Viral covalently closed circular DNA in a non-transgenic mouse model for chronic hepatitis B virus replication. *J Hepatol.* 2006;44:267-274.

[271] Webster GJ, Reignat S, Maini MK, Whalley SA, Ogg GS, King A, Brown D, Amlot PL, Williams R, Vergani D, Dusheiko GM, Bertoletti A. Incubation phase of acute hepatitis B in man: dynamic of cellular immune mechanisms. *Hepatology.* 2000;32:1117-1124.

[272] Maini MK, Boni C, Lee CK, Larrubia JR, Reignat S, Ogg GS, King AS, Herberg J, Gilson R, Alisa A, Williams R, Vergani D, Naoumov NV, Ferrari C, Bertoletti A. The role of virus-specific CD8(+) cells in liver damage and viral control during persistent hepatitis B virus infection. *J Exp Med.* 2000;191:1269-1280.

[273] Nayersina R, Fowler P, Guilhot S, Missale G, Cerny A, Schlicht HJ, Vitiello A, Chesnut R, Person JL, Redeker AG, Chisari FV. HLA A2 restricted cytotoxic T lymphocyte responses to multiple hepatitis B surface antigen epitopes during hepatitis B virus infection. *J Immunol.* 1993;150:4659-4671.

[274] Mehal WZ, Juedes AE and Crispe IN. Selective retention of activated CD8+ T cells by the normal liver. *J Immunol* 1999; 163: 3202-3210.

[275] Kakimi K, Lane TE, Chisari FV, Guidotti LG. Cutting edge: Inhibition of hepatitis B virus replication by activated NK T cells does not require inflammatory cell recruitment to the liver. *J Immunol.* 2001;167:6701-6705.

[276] Zlotnik A, Yoshie O. Chemokines: a new classification system and their role in immunity. *Immunity.* 2000;12:121-127.

[277] Rossi D, Zlotnik A. The biology of chemokines and their receptors. *Annu Rev Immunol.* 2000;18:217-42.

[278] Park JW, Gruys ME, McCormick K, Lee JK, Subleski J, Wigginton JM, Fenton RG, Wang JM, Wiltrout RH. Primary hepatocytes from mice treated with IL-2/IL-12 produce T cell chemoattractant activity that is dependent on monokine induced by IFN-gamma (Mig) and chemokine responsive to gamma-2 (Crg-2). *J Immunol.* 200;166:3763-3770.

[279] Kakimi K, Lane TE, Wieland S, Asensio VC, Campbell IL, Chisari FV, Guidotti LG. Blocking chemokine responsive to gamma-2/interferon (IFN)-gamma inducible protein and monokine induced by IFN-gamma activity in vivo reduces the pathogenetic but not the antiviral potential of hepatitis B virus-specific cytotoxic T lymphocytes. *J Exp Med.* 2001;194:1755-1766.

[280] Sitia G, Isogawa M, Kakimi K, Wieland SF, Chisari FV, Guidotti LG. Depletion of neutrophils blocks the recruitment of antigen-nonspecific cells into the liver without affecting the antiviral activity of hepatitis B virus-specific cytotoxic T lymphocytes. *Proc Natl Acad Sci U S A.* 2002;99:13717-13722.

[281] Scapini P, Lapinet-Vera JA, Gasperini S, Calzetti F, Bazzoni F, Cassatella MA. The neutrophil as a cellular source of chemokines. Immunol Rev. 2000;177:195-203.

[282] Fessler MB, Malcolm KC, Duncan MW, Worthen GS. A genomic and proteomic analysis of activation of the human neutrophil by lipopolysaccharide and its mediation by p38 mitogen-activated protein kinase. *J Biol Chem.* 2002;277:31291-31302.

[283] Vierucci A, De Martino M, Graziani E, Rossi ME, London WT, Blumberg BS. A mechanism for liver cell injury in viral hepatitis: effects of hepatitis B virus on neutrophil function in vitro and in children with chronic active hepatitis. *Pediatr Res.* 1983;17:814-820.

[284] Leifeld L, Cheng S, Ramakers J, Dumoulin FL, Trautwein C, Sauerbruch T, Spengler U. Imbalanced intrahepatic expression of interleukin 12, interferon gamma, and interleukin 10 in fulminant hepatitis B. *Hepatology.* 2002;36:1001-1008.

[285] Nicoletti F, Di Marco R, Zaccone P, Salvaggio A, Magro G, Bendtzen K, Meroni P. Murine concanavalin A-induced hepatitis is prevented by interleukin 12 (IL-12) antibody and exacerbated by exogenous IL-12 through an interferon-gamma-dependent mechanism. *Hepatology.* 2000;32:728-733.

[286] Myers KJ, Eppihimer MJ, Hall L, Wolitzky B. Interleukin-12-induced adhesion molecule expression in murine liver. *Am J Pathol.* 1998;152:457-468.

[287] Sobao Y, Tomiyama H, Sugi K, Tokunaga M, Ueno T, Saito S, Fujiyama S, Morimoto M, Tanaka K, Takiguchi M. The role of hepatitis B virus-specific memory CD8 T cells in the control of viral replication. *J Hepatol.* 2002;36:105-115.

[288] Thimme R, Wieland S, Steiger C, Ghrayeb J, Reimann KA, Purcell RH, Chisari FV. CD8(+) T cells mediate viral clearance and disease pathogenesis during acute hepatitis B virus infection. *J Virol.* 2003;77:68-76.

[289] Shimada N, Yamamoto K, Kuroda MJ, Terada R, Hakoda T, Shimomura H, Hata H, Nakayama E, Shiratori Y. HBcAg-specific CD8 T cells play an important role in virus suppression, and acute flare-up is associated with the expansion of activated memory T cells. *J Clin Immunol.* 2003;23:223-232.

[290] Tang TJ, Kwekkeboom J, Laman JD, Niesters HG, Zondervan PE, de Man RA, Schalm SW, Janssen HL. The role of intrahepatic immune effector cells in inflammatory liver injury and viral control during chronic hepatitis B infection. *J Viral Hepat.* 2003;10:159-167.

[291] Bravo AA, Sheth SG, Chopra S. Liver biopsy. *N Engl J Med.* 2001;344:495-500.

[292] Webster GJ, Reignat S, Brown D, Ogg GS, Jones L, Seneviratne SL, Williams R, Dusheiko G, Bertoletti A. Longitudinal analysis of CD8+ T cells specific for structural and nonstructural hepatitis B virus proteins in patients with chronic hepatitis B: implications for immunotherapy. *J Virol.* 2004;78:5707-5719.

[293] Tang TJ, Janssen HL, Kusters JG, de Man RA, Schalm SW, Kwekkeboom J. The intrahepatic immune response during chronic hepatitis B infection can be monitored by the fine-needle aspiration biopsy technique. *FEMS Immunol Med Microbiol.* 2003;39:69-72.

[294] Sprengers D, van der Molen RG, Kusters JG, De Man RA, Niesters HG, Schalm SW, Janssen HL. Analysis of intrahepatic HBV-specific cytotoxic T-cells during and after acute HBV infection in humans. *J Hepatol.* 2006;45:182-189.

[295] Sprengers D, van der Molen RG, Kusters JG, Kwekkeboom J, van der Laan LJ, Niesters HG, Kuipers EJ, De Man RA, Schalm SW, Janssen HL. Flow cytometry of fine-needle-aspiration biopsies: a new method to monitor the intrahepatic immunological environment in chronic viral hepatitis. *J Viral Hepat.* 2005;12:507-512.

[296] Dunn C, Brunetto M, Reynolds G, Christophides T, Kennedy PT, Lampertico P, Das A, Lopes AR, Borrow P, Williams K, Humphreys E, Afford S, Adams DH, Bertoletti A, Maini MK. Cytokines induced during chronic hepatitis B virus infection promote a pathway for NK cell-mediated liver damage. *J Exp Med.* 2007;204:667-680.

[297] Grakoui A, John Wherry E, Hanson HL, Walker C, Ahmed R. Turning on the off switch: regulation of anti-viral T cell responses in the liver by the PD-1/PD-L1 pathway. *J Hepatol.* 2006;45:468-472.

[298] Muhlbauer M, Fleck M, Schutz C, Weiss T, Froh M, Blank C, Scholmerich J, Hellerbrand C. PD-L1 is induced in hepatocytes by viral infection and by interferon-alpha and -gamma and mediates T cell apoptosis. *J Hepatol.* 2006;45:520-528.

[299] Boni C, Fisicaro P, Valdatta C, Amadei B, Di Vincenzo P, Giuberti T, Laccabue D, Zerbini A, Cavalli A, Missale G, Bertoletti A, Ferrari C. Characterization of Hepatitis B Virus (HBV)-Specific T-Cell Dysfunction in Chronic HBV Infection. *J Virol.* 2007;81:4215-4225.

[300] Kaech SM, Tan JT, Wherry EJ, Konieczny BT, Surh CD, Ahmed R. Selective expression of the interleukin 7 receptor identifies effector CD8 T cells that give rise to long-lived memory cells. *Nat Immunol.* 2003; 4:1191-1198.

[301] Huster KM, Busch V, Schiemann M, Linkemann K, Kerksiek KM, Wagner H, Busch DH. Selective expression of IL-7 receptor on memory T cells identifies early CD40L-dependent generation of distinct CD8+ memory T cell subsets. *Proc Natl Acad Sci U S A.* 2004; 101:5610-5615.

[302] Tebo AE, Fuller MJ, Gaddis DE, Kojima K, Rehani K, Zajac AJ. Rapid recruitment of virus-specific CD8 T cells restructures immunodominance during protective secondary responses. *J Virol.* 2005;79:12703-12713.

[303] Bachmann MF, Wolint P, Schwarz K, Oxenius A. Recall proliferation potential of memory CD8+ T cells and antiviral protection. *J Immunol.* 2005;175:4677-4685.

[304] Lang KS, Recher M, Navarini AA, Harris NL, Lohning M, Junt T, Probst HC, Hengartner H, Zinkernagel RM. Inverse correlation between IL-7 receptor expression and CD8 T cell exhaustion during persistent antigen stimulation. *Eur J Immunol.* 2005;35:738-745.

[305] Boettler T, Panther E, Bengsch B, Nazarova N, Spangenberg HC, Blum HE, Thimme R. Expression of the interleukin-7 receptor alpha chain (CD127) on virus-specific CD8+ T cells identifies functionally and phenotypically defined memory T cells during acute resolving hepatitis B virus infection. *J Virol.* 2006;80:3532-3540.

[306] Day CL, Kaufmann DE, Kiepiela P, Brown JA, Moodley ES, Reddy S, Mackey EW, Miller JD, Leslie AJ, DePierres C, Mncube Z, Duraiswamy J, Zhu B, Eichbaum Q, Altfeld M, Wherry EJ, Coovadia HM, Goulder PJ, Klenerman P, Ahmed R, Freeman GJ, Walker BD. PD-1 expression on HIV-specific T cells is associated with T-cell exhaustion and disease progression. *Nature.* 2006;443:350-354.

[307] Zhang JY, Zhang Z, Wang X, Fu JL, Yao J, Jiao Y, Chen L, Zhang H, Wei J, Jin L, Shi M, Gao GF, Wu H, Wang FS. PD-1 upregulation is correlated with HIV-specific memory CD8+ T-cell exhaustion in typical progressors, but not in long-term non-progressors. *Blood.* 2007 Feb 1;

[308] Cai G, Karni A, Oliveira EM, Weiner HL, Hafler DA, Freeman GJ. PD-1 ligands, negative regulators for activation of naive, memory, and recently activated human CD4+ T cells. *Cell Immunol.* 2004;230:89-98.

[309] Gehring AJ, Sun D, Kennedy PT, Nolte-'t Hoen E, Lim SG, Wasser S, Selden C, Maini MK, Davis DM, Nassal M, Bertoletti A. The level of viral antigen presented by hepatocytes influences CD8 T-cell function. *J Virol.* 2007;81:2940-2949.

[310] Isogawa M, Furuichi Y, Chisari FV.Oscillating CD8(+) T cell effector functions after antigen recognition in the liver. *Immunity.* 2005;23:53-63.

[311] Hoofnagle JH, Doo E, Liang TJ, Fleischer R, Lok AS. Management of hepatitis B: summary of a clinical research workshop. *Hepatology.* 2007;45:1056-1075.

[312] Tillmann HL. Antiviral therapy and resistance with hepatitis B virus infection. *World J Gastroenterol.* 2007;13:125-140.

[313] Boni C, Bertoletti A, Penna A, Cavalli A, Pilli M, Urbani S, Scognamiglio P, Boehme R, Panebianco R, Fiaccadori F, Ferrari C. Lamivudine treatment can restore T cell responsiveness in chronic hepatitis B. *J Clin Invest.* 1998;102:968-975.

[314] Boni C, Penna A, Ogg GS, Bertoletti A, Pilli M, Cavallo C, Cavalli A, Urbani S, Boehme R, Panebianco R, Fiaccadori F, Ferrari C. Lamivudine treatment can overcome cytotoxic T-cell hyporesponsiveness in chronic hepatitis B: new perspectives for immune therapy. *Hepatology.* 2001;33:963-971.

[315] Boni C, Penna A, Bertoletti A, Lamonaca V, Rapti I, Missale G, Pilli M, Urbani S, Cavalli A, Cerioni S, Panebianco R, Jenkins J, Ferrari C. Transient restoration of anti-viral T cell responses induced by lamivudine therapy in chronic hepatitis B. *J Hepatol.* 2003;39:595-605.

[316] Malacarne F, Webster GJ, Reignat S, Gotto J, Behboudi S, Burroughs AK, Dusheiko GM, Williams R, Bertoletti A. Tracking the source of the hepatitis B virus-specific CD8 T cells during lamivudine treatment. *J Infect Dis.* 2003;187:679-682.

[317] Tang TJ, de Man RA, Kusters JG, Kwekkeboom J, Hop WC, van der Molen RG, Schalm SW, Janssen HL. Intrahepatic CD8 T-lymphocytes and HBV core expression in relation to response to antiviral therapy for chronic hepatitis B patients. *J Med Virol.* 2004;72:215-222.

[318] Tang TJ, Kwekkeboom J, Mancham S, Binda RS, de Man RA, Schalm SW, Kusters JG, Janssen HL. Intrahepatic CD8+ T-lymphocyte response is important for therapy-induced viral clearance in chronic hepatitis B infection. *J Hepatol.* 2005;43:45-52.

[319] Lin CL, Tsai SL, Lee TH, Chien RN, Liao SK, Liaw YF. High frequency of functional anti-YMDD and -mutant cytotoxic T lymphocytes after in vitro expansion correlates with successful response to lamivudine therapy for chronic hepatitis B. *Gut.* 2005;54:152-161.

[320] van der Molen RG, Sprengers D, Biesta PJ, Kusters JG, Janssen HL. Favorable effect of adefovir on the number and functionality of myeloid dendritic cells of patients with chronic HBV. *Hepatology.* 2006;44:907-914.

[321] Stoop JN, van der Molen RG, Kuipers EJ, Kusters JG, Janssen HL. Inhibition of viral replication reduces regulatory T cells and enhances the antiviral immune response in chronic hepatitis B. *Virology.* 2007;361:141-148.

[322] Riordan SM, Skinner N, Kurtovic J, Locarnini S, Visvanathan K. Reduced expression of toll-like receptor 2 on peripheral monocytes in patients with chronic hepatitis B. *Clin Vaccine Immunol.* 2006;13:972-974.

[323] Alcami A, Koszinowski UH. Viral mechanisms of immune evasion. *Mol Med Today.* 2000;6:365-372.

[324] Hilleman MR. Strategies and mechanisms for host and pathogen survival in acute and persistent viral infections. Proc Natl Acad Sci U S A. 2004;101 *Suppl* 2:14560-14566.

[325] Gewurz BE, Gaudet R, Tortorella D, Wang EW, Ploegh HL. Virus subversion of immunity: a structural perspective. *Curr Opin Immunol.* 2001;13:442-450.

[326] Umeda M, Marusawa H, Seno H, Katsurada A, Nabeshima M, Egawa H, Uemoto S, Inomata Y, Tanaka K, Chiba T. Hepatitis B virus infection in lymphatic tissues in inactive hepatitis B carriers. *J Hepatol.* 2005;42:806-812.

[327] Dejean A, Lugassy C, Zafrani S, Tiollais P, Brechot C. Detection of hepatitis B virus DNA in pancreas, kidney and skin of two human carriers of the virus. *J Gen Virol.* 1984;65:651-655.

[328] Torresi J. The virological and clinical significance of mutations in the overlapping envelope and polymerase genes of hepatitis B virus. *J Clin Virol.* 2002;25:97-106.

[329] Torresi J, Earnest-Silveira L, Deliyannis G, Edgtton K, Zhuang H, Locarnini SA, Fyfe J, Sozzi T, Jackson DC. Reduced antigenicity of the hepatitis B virus HBsAg protein arising as a consequence of sequence changes in the overlapping polymerase gene that are selected by lamivudine therapy. *Virology.* 2002;293:305-313.

[330] Lu HY, Zeng Z, Xu XY, Zhang NL, Yu M, Gong WB. Mutations in surface and polymerase gene of chronic hepatitis B patients with coexisting HBsAg and anti-HBs. *World J Gastroenterol.* 2006;12:4219-4223.

[331] Pircher H, Moskophidis D, Rohrer U, Burki K, Hengartner H, Zinkernagel RM. Viral escape by selection of cytotoxic T cell-resistant virus variants in vivo. *Nature.* 1990;346:629-633.

[332] Michalak TI, Hodgson PD, Churchill ND. Posttranscriptional inhibition of class I major histocompatibility complex presentation on hepatocytes and lymphoid cells in chronic woodchuck hepatitis virus infection. *J Virol.* 2000;74:4483-4494.

[333] Maini MK, Reignat S, Boni C, Ogg GS, King AS, Malacarne F, Webster GJ, Bertoletti A. T cell receptor usage of virus-specific CD8 cells and recognition of viral mutations during acute and persistent hepatitis B virus infection. *Eur J Immunol.* 2000;30:3067-3078.

[334] Khakoo SI, Ling R, Scott I, Dodi AI, Harrison TJ, Dusheiko GM, Madrigal JA. Cytotoxic T lymphocyte responses and CTL epitope escape mutation in HBsAg, anti-HBe positive individuals. *Gut.* 2000;47:137-143.

[335] Carman WF, Boner W, Fattovich G, Colman K, Dornan ES, Thursz M, Hadziyannis S. protein mutations are concentrated in B cell epitopes in progressive disease and in T helper cell epitopes during clinical remission. *J Infect Dis.* 1997;175:1093-1100.

[336] Lee YI, Hur GM, Suh DJ, Kim SH. Novel pre-C/C gene mutants of hepatitis B virus in chronic active hepatitis: naturally occurring escape mutants. *J Gen Virol.* 1996;77:1129-1138.

[337] Kato J, Hasegawa K, Torii N, Yamauchi K, Hayashi N. A molecular analysis of viral persistence in surface antigen-negative chronic hepatitis B. *Hepatology.* 1996;23:389-395.

[338] Protzer-Knolle U, Naumann U, Bartenschlager R, Berg T, Hopf U, Meyer zum Buschenfelde KH, Neuhaus P, Gerken G. Hepatitis B virus with antigenically altered hepatitis B surface antigen is selected by high-dose hepatitis B immune globulin after liver transplantation. *Hepatology.* 1998;27:254-263.

[339] van der Molen RG, Sprengers D, Binda RS, de Jong EC, Niesters HG, Kusters JG, Kwekkeboom J, Janssen HL. Functional impairment of myeloid and plasmacytoid dendritic cells of patients with chronic hepatitis. *Hepatology.* 2004;40:738-746.

[340] Rossol S, Marinos G, Carucci P, Singer MV, Williams R, Naoumov NV. Interleukin-12 induction of Th1 cytokines is important for viral clearance in chronic hepatitis B. *J Clin Invest.* 1997;99:3025-3033.

[341] Kimura K, Kakimi K, Wieland S, Guidotti LG, Chisari FV. Activated intrahepatic antigen-presenting cells inhibit hepatitis B virus replication in the liver of transgenic mice. *J Immunol.* 2002;169:5188-5195.

[342] Wherry EJ, Blattman JN, Murali-Krishna K, van der Most R, Ahmed R. Viral persistence alters CD8 T-cell immunodominance and tissue distribution and results in distinct stages of functional impairment. *J Virol.* 2003;77:4911-4927.

[343] Brooks DG, Teyton L, Oldstone MB, McGavern DB. Intrinsic functional dysregulation of CD4 T cells occurs rapidly following persistent viral infection. *J Virol.* 2005;79:10514-10527.

[344] Moskophidis D, Lechner F, Pircher H, Zinkernagel RM. Virus persistence in acutely infected immunocompetent mice by exhaustion of antiviral cytotoxic effector T cells. *Nature.* 1993;362:758-761.

[345] Ploegh HL. Viral strategies of immune evasion. *Science.* 1998;280:248-253.

[346] Reignat S, Webster GJ, Brown D, Ogg GS, King A, Seneviratne SL, Dusheiko G, Williams R, Maini MK, Bertoletti A. Escaping high viral load exhaustion: CD8 cells with altered tetramer binding in chronic hepatitis B virus infection. *J Exp Med.* 2002;195:1089-1101.

[347] Urbani S, Amadei B, Fisicaro P, Tola D, Orlandini A, Sacchelli L, Mori C, Missale G, Ferrari C. Outcome of acute hepatitis C is related to virus-specific CD4 function and maturation of antiviral memory CD8 responses. *Hepatology.* 2006;44:126-139.

[348]   Zajac AJ, Blattman JN, Murali-Krishna K, Sourdive DJ, Suresh M,
        Altman JD, Ahmed R. Viral immune evasion due to persistence of
        activated T cells without effector function. *J Exp Med.* 1998;188:2205-
        2213.

[349]   Tuttleman JS, Pourcel C, Summers J. Formation of the pool of covalently
        closed circular viral DNA in hepadnavirus-infected cells. *Cell.*
        1986;47:451-460.

[350]   Stoop JN, van der Molen RG, Baan CC, van der Laan LJ, Kuipers EJ,
        Kusters JG, Janssen HL Regulatory T cells contribute to the impaired
        immune response in patients with chronic hepatitis B virus infection.
        Hepatology. 2005;41:771-778.

[351]   Franzese O, Kennedy PT, Gehring AJ, Gotto J, Williams R, Maini MK,
        Bertoletti A. Modulation of the CD8+-T-cell response by CD4+ CD25+
        regulatory T cells in patients with hepatitis B virus infection. *J Virol.*
        2005;79:3322-3328.

[352]   Kondo Y, Kobayashi K, Ueno Y, Shiina M, Niitsuma H, Kanno N,
        Kobayashi T, Shimosegawa T. Mechanism of T cell hyporesponsiveness
        to HBcAg is associated with regulatory T cells in chronic hepatitis B.
        World J Gastroenterol. 2006;12:4310-4317.

[353]   Moore KW, de Waal Malefyt R, Coffman RL, O'Garra A. Interleukin-10
        and the interleukin-10 receptor. *Annu Rev Immunol.* 2001;19:683-765.

[354]   Miyazoe S, Hamasaki K, Nakata K, Kajiya Y, Kitajima K, Nakao K,
        Daikoku M, Yatsuhashi H, Koga M, Yano M, Eguchi K. Influence of
        interleukin-10 gene promoter polymorphisms on disease progression in
        patients chronically infected with hepatitis B virus. *Am J Gastroenterol.*
        2002;97:2086-2092.

[355]   Harari A, Vallelian F, Pantaleo G. Phenotypic heterogeneity of antigen-
        specific CD4 T cells under different conditions of antigen persistence and
        antigen load. *Eur J Immunol.* 2004;34:3525-3533.

[356]   Sallusto F, Geginat J, Lanzavecchia A.Central memory and effector
        memory T cell subsets: function, generation, and maintenance. *Annu Rev
        Immunol.* 2004;22:745-763.

Authors' Affiliations

Sirio Fiorino[1,2], Ranka Vukotic[2], Elisabetta Loggi[2], Giovanni Vitale[2], Carmela Cursaro[2], Cinzia Fortini[2], Annagiulia Gramenzi[2], Lorenzo Micco[2], Andrea Cuppini[1], Mauro Bernardi[2], Pietro Andreone[2].

[1] U.O. Medicina Interna Ospedale di Budrio. Azienda Unità Sanitaria Locale di Bologna. Italy.

[2] Dipartimento di Medicina Interna, Cardioangiologia, Epatologia. University of Bologna. Bologna. Italy.

Corresponding Author:
Pietro Andreone, MD
Address:
Dipartimento di Medicina Interna, Cardioangiologia, Epatologia -Università di Bologna
Policlinico S.Orsola-Malpighi
via Massarenti 9,
40138 Bologna (ITALY)
e-mail: andreone@med.unibo.it
phone: +39.051.6363871
fax: +39.051.345806

Index

H

I

R

S

T

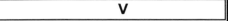